Disease, Drugs, an

Disease, Drugs, and the Dentist

by

HUMPHREY D. ASTLEY HOPE MB., BS., BDS., D.Orth.

General Dental Practitioner and Dental Surgeon to Newbury District Hospital

and

MICHAEL D. HELLIER MA., MB., Bch., FRCP., MD.

Consultant Physician Princess Margaret Hospital, Swindon

A Wiley Medical Publication

JOHN WILEY & SONS

Chichester · New York · Brisbane · Toronto · Singapore

Library of Congress Cataloging in Publication Data:

Astley Hope, Humphrey D.
Disease, drugs, and the dentist.

(A Wiley medical publication)
Includes index.
1. Dentistry, Operative—Complications and sequelae.
2. Diseases—Complications and sequelae. 3. Chemotherapy—Complications and sequelae. I. Hellier, Michael D. II. Title.
III. Series. [DNLM: 1. Disease—Handbooks. 2. Drug Therapy—Handbooks. 3. Dentistry—Handbooks. WU 100 H79ld]
RK513.A87 1983 617.6 82-11175
ISBN 0 471 90016-8 AACR2

British Library Cataloguing in Publication Data:

Astley Hope, Humphrey D.
Disease, drugs, and the dentist.
1. Periodontics
I. Title II. Hellier, Michael D.
617.6′3206 RK361

ISBN 0 471 90016 8
Printed by the Pitman Press Ltd., Bath, Avon.

Contents

Preface

Section 1

Alphabetical List of Diseases and Conditions 1

Section 2

Alphabetical list of Pharmacological and Proprietary Drug Names 223

Preface

This little book is written as an 'aide memoire', primarily for the general dental practitioner. In no way should it be considered as a textbook of Oral Medicine or even a manual of Oral Signs of General Disease. It is designed to assist the dentist when confronted with a patient who tells him/her that he suffers from a certain condition and is under treatment with such and such a drug.

The contents have been laid out alphabetically in two sections. The first lists diseases and conditions likely to be encountered, and the second drugs which the patient may be taking. The former are given under their proper (medical) titles, with their colloquial names cross-referenced to them. The drugs in the latter section are set out under their pharmacological titles with proprietary names (GB and US) similarly cross-referenced. For the sake of brevity the lists are far from complete. Primary diseases of the teeth and gums have been omitted, as it was felt that the readers would be as conversant with these as the authors. The selection is based on three principles; firstly, diseases of which the sufferers may be at hazard in the course of dental treatment either by reason of the disease itself or its treatment; secondly, communicable diseases where special precautions should be taken to protect dentist, staff, and other patients; and lastly, a general group with or without oral manifestations, whose names may crop up in taking a medical history.

As in other books of this type, a number of statements are based on the opinion of the authors and are not substantiated by proof. As an example, we advise the use of a local anaesthetic without adrenaline in patients with certain cardiovascular conditions. Research has not demonstrated any dangerous rise in blood adrenaline following the extravascular injection of a local anaesthetic with adrenaline in reasonable quantity. However, aspirating syringes are only as foolproof as the hand that holds them, and, while the effects of intravenous prilocaine and felypressin on a damaged human heart have not been investigated, we feel that this alternative or lignocaine alone would be less dangerous than a local anaesthetic containing adrenaline under these circumstances.

The authors have done their best to supply United States equivalents of drugs used in Great Britain, but in a few instances no equivalent is listed, and, no doubt, there are other situations where a drug is used in the United States and not here. In such a wide and complex field, there will be omissions and errors resulting from recent study with which we are unacquainted, but we hope these are not of sufficient magnitude to seriously mislead a dentist consulting the book for guidance.

An index and list of references have been omitted to conserve space, but readers are advised to refer to standard textbooks of General and Dental Medicine in situations where they wish to find out more about the subject.

The authors wish to thank professional colleagues whom they have consulted during the preparation of this book, particularly Professor W.H. Binnie of Baylor College of Dentistry, Dallas; Mr John Fieldhouse of the Department of Oral Surgery, Princess Margaret Hospital, Swindon and Dr Patrick Smythe of St John's Road, Newbury. We acknowledge with gratitude advice and assistance from Dr John Jarvis of John Wiley & Sons on the presentation of the script. Both of us owe a great debt to our secretaries, Mrs Jacqueline Birch, Miss Sharon Brain, and Mrs Doreen Burnup who have coped uncomplaining with sheaves of barely legible handwriting, and to our two patient wives who have supplied both material help and encouragement.

In conclusion we should like to thank Professor Brian Cooke, Dean of the Dental School, University of Wales whose suggestion initiated this book and who checked through our manuscripts at the end. It might be said that he abetted procreation and was midwife to delivery.

SECTION 1

Alphabetical List of Diseases and Conditions

A

ACHALASIA

This is a disturbance of the swallowing mechanism due to denervation of the lower oesophagus, which is unable to relax during swallowing. The oesophageal musculature above this level hypertrophies and the oesophagus progressively dilates. The aetiology is unknown. As the condition progresses food accumulates in the oesophagus and putrefies. The mucosa becomes inflamed, and in approximately 5 per cent of people, carcinoma of oesophagus occurs. A more common complication is lung aspiration with progressive pulmonary disease. The condition occurs in either sex, at any age. Pain is a frequent presenting feature, sometimes mimicking angina and occurs in 80 per cent of people. Dysphagia and regurgitation, often of foul-smelling food remnants, become progressively more severe and are accompanied by weight loss.

The diagnosis is made by barium swallow. Drug treatment has little to offer, although occasional inhalation of **octyl nitrate** can relieve the pain of oesophageal spasm.

The treatment of choice is surgery. The circular muscle layer of the lower oesophagus is cut (Heller's operation). Alternative treatment is rupture of the circular muscle layer by balloon dilatation.

Dental Significance

Because regurgitation of solid matter can occur many hours after the last meal, general anaesthesia is a hazard. If essential for dental treatment, it should be carried out by intubation with a cuffed tube. The possibility of underlying lung disease must be borne in mind. Achalasia should be remembered as a cause of halitosis when no oral or pulmonary disease is present to account for it.

ACHONDROPLASIA

This hereditary failure in the ossification of bones formed in cartilage, appears in foetal life. Those who survive are the circus dwarfs with short limbs and large heads. There is no treatment, but apart from the bone deformity health and life expectation is normal.

Dental Significance

Growth of the mandible is unaffected but that of the middle third of the face is deficient. This results in a Class III malocclusion but the teeth themselves are usually normal. Intubation can be difficult, if required for general anaesthesia.

ACNE VULGARIS

This condition commences at puberty and is due to over-activity of the sebaceous glands. The main distribution is on the face, central chest, and back, the areas of highest sebum production. The sex incidence is equal. Hyperkeratosis and inspissation of sebum in the follicles cause the primary lesion of acne, the comedone or blackhead. An inflammatory response may produce sterile pus forming a pustule.

Mild peeling agents such as sulphur and salicylic acid are useful treatment. **Benzoyl peroxide** as a cream or lotion may be beneficial. Long-term use of antibiotics by mouth may be very effective, **tetracycline** being the antibiotic of choice. Exposure on a regular basis to ultraviolet light, either natural or by lamp, is advocated.

Dental Significance

None.

ACRODERMATITIS ENTEROPATHICA

This is a persistent dermatitis affecting the perioral area and peripheries, commencing with vesicles which progress to crusting, thickening, and sometimes secondary infection. Two-thirds of patients have a family history. Plasma zinc levels are low and the condition responds dramatically to treatment with zinc supplements. It may be confused with psoriasis or candidiasis.

Dental Significance

Oedema, desquamation, and ulceration of the oral mucosa may be seen in addition to weeping erosions at the corners of the mouth. The condition is not infectious.

ACROMEGALY

Excess of growth hormone, which in young life results in gigantism, causes acromegaly after the epiphyses have closed. It is produced by an acidophil tumour of the anterior pituitary gland. A large jaw, coarse skin, and spade-like hands are the special features. Muscle weakness, defective vision, and diabetes are not uncommon.

Treatment is by surgical removal of the tumour or irradiation. **Bromocriptine** is used to suppress high levels of growth hormone.

Dental Significance

The skeletal discrepancies between maxilla and mandible are gross and any correction, after eradication of the tumour, will require surgery.

General anaesthetics should only be administered in hospital, and, even then, not entertained lightly. Apart from the incidence of diabetes mellitus and other defects, the physical deformity of the mouth can make intubation very difficult.

ACTINOMYCOSIS

This rare bacterial infection, which occurs chiefly in males between 20 and 30, affects the body in one of three sites: the cervicofacial area, the ileocaecal part of intestines, or the lungs. In each it produces a hard mass of tissue which eventually breaks down and discharges through multiple sinuses.

It is treated by high doses of **penicillin** over a long period and by surgery.

Dental Significance

The cervicofacial area is the commonest site, where the condition usually presents as a hard nodular swelling at the angle of the jaw. The skin which is bound to it is blue–red and multiple sinuses develop discharging pus which may show to the naked eye the characteristic yellow granules. There is often trismus. Bone involvement is rare unless there has been a recent fracture or extraction, and the lymph glands are seldom swollen without secondary infection.

Microscopical examination of the pus will usually show the pseudo-mycelium of the bacteria and clinch the diagnosis.

ADDISON'S DISEASE, see ADRENAL DISEASES.

ADRENAL DISEASES

The adrenal gland is composed of an outer cortex and central medulla. The cortex secretes the following hormones:

(1) mineralocorticoids, mainly aldosterone;
(2) glucocorticoids, cortisol, and corticosterone;
(3) androgens, and to a lesser extent progesterone and oestrone.

The medulla produces two hormones:

(1) adrenaline;
(2) nor-adrenaline.

The following conditions result from over-activity of the adrenal gland:

(1) Cushing's syndrome;
(2) primary hyperaldosteronism (Conn's syndrome);
(3) phaeochromocytoma;

and from under-activity:

(1) Addison's disease.

CUSHING'S SYNDROME

This condition results from over-activity of the adrenal cortex and may be due to hyperplasia, or to benign or malignant tumours. The features of the condition are due to excessive glucocorticoid production, causing obesity with a characteristic distribution of fat over the neck and trunk but sparing the arms and legs. The face becomes rounded with a high colour. Acne, hirsutism, and amenorrhoea occur in women, and impotence in men. Other symptoms include weakness, bruising, backache, and symptoms of the complications of Cushing's syndrome, hypertension, diabetes, and depression. The treatment of an adenoma or carcinoma is surgical. Treatment of bilateral adrenal hyperplasia is controversial and may be surgical, adrenalectomy with or without pituitary irradiation and hormone replacement. Medical adrenalectomy may be produced with certain enzyme-blocking drugs.

Patients who have been treated by adrenalectomy will be on a maintenance dose of cortisone. This will require supplementing for surgery (see next section ADDISON'S DISEASE).

PRIMARY HYPERALDOSTERONISM (Conn's syndrome)

This condition results from a defect in the adrenal cortex leading to increased aldosterone production and resulting in hypertension and hypo-kalaemia. The latter may produce muscle weakness, paraesthesia, tetany, polyuria, and thirst.

Treatment may be surgical with adrenalectomy, or medical using aldosterone antagonists.

PHAEOCHROMOCYTOMA

This is a tumour of the adrenal medulla producing excessive quantities of adrenaline and nor-adrenaline. This causes paroxysmal or persistent hypertension. In the paroxysmal type the patient may describe episodes when he or she experiences a feeling of apprehension, palpitations, excessive sweating, flushing, epigastric fulness, and headaches. Treatment where possible is surgical with removal of the tumour. If this is not possible, for example an inoperable malignant tumour, hypertension is controlled with alpha- and beta-adrenergic blocking drugs.

Dental Significance

Dental treatment of patients with over-activity of the adrenal glands must be approached with caution. Hypertension and blood vessel fragility increases the danger of bruising and haemorrhage following surgery. Osteoporosis weakens the bones and fracture of the maxillary tuberosity or the mandible can occur at the time of extractions. Diabetes is an added complication (see DIABETES MELLITUS). General anaesthetics are to be avoided or given in hospital.

ADDISON'S DISEASE

This condition most commonly results from autoimmune adrenalitis or tuberculosis. The clinical features result from loss of cortisol and aldosterone. The condition is more common in women than men and may have been present for years before the diagnosis is made. The prevalence is approximately 1 in 25,000 of the population. The main signs and symptoms are tiredness, weakness, anorexia, and nausea. Pigmentation due to excess adrenocorticotrophin (ACTH) production is characteristic, being prominent inside the cheeks, on the gums and lips. Vomiting, weight loss, dizziness, and postural hypotension are other common features.

Of great importance is the fact that patients with Addison's may be asymptomatic until stressed by intercurrent illness when they may become acutely ill with vomiting and severe hypotension (Addisonian crisis).

Treatment is with **cortisone**, usually 20 mg in the morning and 10 mg at night.

Major surgery requires parenteral treatment, 100 mg **hydrocortisone succinate** IM every 6 hours, starting with the pre-medication and continuing for 72 hours or until the patient is able to take cortisone by mouth. The above procedure also applies to minor surgery but followed for 24 hours only. Very minor procedures may be covered by 100 mg **hydrocortisone succinate** IM.

Treatment of Adrenal Crisis

In this serious event 100 mg **hydrocortisone** IM should be given immediately and an intravenous infusion established, with a further 100 mg **hydrocortisone** given IV. One litre of normal saline plus 50 g **glucose** is given intravenously over ½ hour, followed by 2–4 litres over 24 hours. 100 mg **hydrocortisone** IV is given every 4 hours.

Dental Significance

Brown patches on the buccal mucosa and gingiva in non-pigmented races may be the first indication of Addison's disease, and should be reported.

At least 200 mg of **hydrocortisone** for injection should be carried in every dental surgery. It should be checked frequently to make sure it is not out of date, and dental assistants should be taught how to mix and prepare it for injection.

Patients with adrenocortical insufficiency, being treated with **cortisone** will require additional **cortisone** when surgery or general anaesthetics are contemplated. If no more than a simple extraction under local anaesthesia, it is sufficient for the patient to double the morning dose of **cortisone, hydrocortisone** by injection being readily available (100 mg intravenously) should there be any evidence of hypotensive collapse. General anaesthetics and more extensive surgery are best carried out in hospital under controlled replacement therapy as described.

Adrenal Insufficiency

If within the previous 12 months any patients have been treated with **cortisone** in excess of 5 mg daily for more than a week, subsequent adrenocortical insufficiency must be suspected. With approval of their doctor they should be given **prednisolone** 5 mg TDS for 2 days starting the day prior to surgery and then the dosage reduced by 5 mg a day over the following 3 days. Soluble **hydrocortisone** must be available.

AGAMMAGLOBULINAEMIA

A wide variety of immunodeficiency disorders are now recognized. X-linked infantile agammaglobulinaemia (Bruton type) is a disease in which B-lymphocytes and plasma cells are absent, resulting in gross deficiency of immunoglobulins. Cell-mediated immunity is normal. This deficiency results in recurrent infections to which there is minimal resistance with consequent rapid spread of infection if untreated. Response to appropriate antibiotics is usually good. Treatment of Bruton type and other immunodeficiencies involves early detection and intensive treatment of infective episodes and injections of gammaglobulin at frequent intervals.

Dental Significance

Strict attention to oral hygiene is of utmost importance. Extractions must be carried out under antibiotic cover.

AGRANULOCYTOSIS AND NEUTROPENIA

Neutropenia is a reduction of white blood cells below the level of 2500/mm^3. Agranulocytosis is complete or almost complete absence of neutrophils. The causes are multiple and include drugs, leukaemias, aplastic anaemia, and hyposplenism.

multiple and include drugs, leukaemias, aplastic anaemia, and hyposplenism.

In practice symptoms are uncommon with a count of 1000–1500/mm^3 and common below 500/mm^3.

ACUTE NEUTROPENIA

Symptoms vary in their severity depending on the acuteness of onset. They may be divided into:

(1) Constitutional symptoms, chills, sweats, headaches, muscle pains, and exhaustion.
(2) Infective symptoms due to invasion of the mucous membranes and skin by bacteria. Lesions in the mouth are most prominent, sore throats, reddening of the throat, progressing to ulceration and mucosal necrosis. Ulcers occur on the gums, lips, buccal mucous membranes, throat, and pharynx. The ulcers are often extremely painful. Necrotic ulceration of the skin also occurs.

CHRONIC NEUTROPENIA

(1) Constitutional symptoms are less severe (infections frequently involve the skin). Fatigue, lassitude, and weakness may be independent of any infection or anaemia.
(2) Infectious symptoms. Recurrent infections are the dominant feature of chronic neutropenia, being prolonged, slow-healing, and resistant to treatment. Infections of the mouth and throat and more common.

Treatment involves prevention, and management of established neutropenia where possible, e.g. withdrawal of causative drug and treatment of complications with appropriate antibiotic therapy.

In the chronic form treatment mainly involves prevention and treatment of infection.

Dental Significance

Recurrent ulcerative and haemorrhagic gingivitis, often associated with destructive periodontal disease, may be the first sign of this condition, and a patient seen with these manifestations should be referred for a white blood cell count without delay. Surgery should be put off if possible, but if extractions are unavoidable they must be carried out under strict antibiotic cover.

ALCAPTONURIA

This is a rare hereditary disorder resulting from the absence of the enzyme homogentisic acid oxidase. Because of this defect homogentisic acid accumulates in cartilage, connective tissue, and urine, giving rise to a degenerative arthritis of the spine and larger peripheral joints.

Dental Significance

Pigmentation of the teeth has been reported.

ALCOHOLISM

An alcoholic may be considered an individual who habitually drinks an excessive amount of alcohol or who has special problems relating to consumption of alcohol. Not all alcoholics develop the medical complications of alcohol and conversely alcohol-induced disease may occur in non-alcoholics.

Addiction is the stage of physical dependence on alcohol and leads to disintegration of social status and personality. Symptoms include memory blanks following drinking sessions, restlessness if without alcohol, tremor, morning retching, vomiting, and night sweating. Cessation of alcohol results in the withdrawal syndromes. The early stage (6–8 hours) includes tremulousness, nausea, retching, and sweating. The late stage (after 48 hours) is the syndrome of delirium tremens, that is mental confusion, disorientation, restlessness, fear, paranoia, hallucinations, and occasionally epilepsy.

Opinions vary as to the dangerous level of daily alcohol intake but most authorities agree that a sustained level of 10–15 units a day in men and 7–10 units in females (where a unit is equivalent to half a pint of beer or a glass of wine) is liable to lead to serious physical harm. However, considerable individual variation in susceptibility to alcohol damage exists.

The physical consequences of alcohol are legion. Accidents commonly result from intoxication and head trauma is frequent. Acute pancreatitis with a high mortality rate complicates high alcohol intake, also gastritis and gastric erosions which may result in haematemesis. There is an increased risk of vascular disease, cardiomyopathy, and tendency to a rise in blood pressure. Liver damage is the best-known complicaton of alcohol abuse. Initially changes are reversible but once cirrhosis is established the damage persists and progresses accompanied by the fearsome complications of portal hypertension, variceal haemorrhage and carcinoma of the liver. Apart from the psychoses associated with alcohol withdrawal, alcohol causes cerebral atrophy, dementia, Korsakoff's psychosis, and Wernicke's encephalopathy. Malnutrition in association with high alcohol consumption may result in wet and dry beri-beri. Peripheral neuropathy occurs in 10 per cent and suicides are much commoner amongst alcoholics.

Treatment. Prevention is of greatest importance for once alcoholism is established very few alcoholics are ever cured. At-risk groups need identifying and advising. Management of the addict includes management of the physical problems and withdrawal syndromes together with techniques to promote abstinence. 'Drying out' is often best carried out in hospital. Promotion of abstinence necessitates a change in attitude best brought about by the help of self-help groups such as 'AA' (Alcoholics Anonymous) and hospital self-help groups. At-risk occupations such as barman or publican should be changed. Living in a therapeutic community such as a hostel for alcoholics may help. Drugs such as **disulfiram** (*Antabuse*)$_{\mathrm{GB,US}}$ have only a limited part to play.

Dental Significance

Most dentists will be more than familiar with the smell of alcohol on the breath and know that even in mid-morning this is not diagnostic of an alcoholic. Any oral manifestations of alcoholism result from associated vitamin deficiency, and are likely to include glossitis, angular cheilitis, and sometimes candida infection and leukoplakia. **Aspirin** is liable to cause gastric irritation, and **paracetamol** should be prescribed as an alternative analgesic, but avoiding large doses. Because of the possibility of incipient liver damage narcotic analgesics and hypnotics should be avoided and **diazepam** (*Valium*)$_{\mathrm{GB,US}}$ used in reduced dosage. **Penicillin** is the safest antibiotic. General anaesthetics are a hazard, and **lignocaine** should be used with restraint.

Oral carcinoma is said to be more common in alcoholics, and the floor of the mouth should be carefully examined for this.

ALLERGIC RHINITIS

This condition, popularly called hay fever, results from allergy to one of the grass pollens or to a multitude of other allergens such as household dust, feathers, or fur. Densensitizing injections prior to its occurrence are often successful when the condition is seasonal or the allergen can be identified. In an attack antihistamines such as **chlorpheniramine** (*Piriton*)$_{GB}$ 4 mg BD, are helpful, but some suit individuals better than others. Nebulizers containing **sodium cromoglycate** (*Rynacrom*)$_{GB}$ or **beclomethasone** (*Beconase*)$_{GB}$ are also of value.

Dental Significance

When possible dentistry should be avoided during attacks. The nasal obstruction is a complicating factor to general anaesthetics and, for sufferers, these are best planned for when the condition is not prevalent. If a general anaesthetic is necessary at short notice, the patient's doctor should be consulted with regards to a short course of **cortisone** (**cortisone acetate** 10 mg TDS) to suppress the symptoms.

ALZHEIMER'S DISEASE

The cause of this rapidly progressive pre-senile dementia is obscure, but it may result from a defect in the earliest stage of protein synthesis. Widespread neuronal degeneration produces an appearance of the cell known as neurofibrillary tangle. Earliest signs are loss of short-term memory followed by inability to reason, impairment of speech, intellect failure, inability to read, increasing helplessness, and death in about 5 years. There is no specific treatment.

Dental Significance

Fortunately rare, this miserable disease is quite as distressing for relatives as it is for its victims. The dentist should be aware of its name and nature to save the embarrassment of explanations. Treatment must be adjusted to that with which the patient can co-operate, bearing in mind the prognosis.

AMYLOIDOSIS

This is the name given to a group of conditions where protein/polysaccharide complexes are laid down in tissue. These may be divided into two main groups:

(1) Primary amyloid, associated with plasma cell dyscrasia and overt myeloma, affecting predominantly the tongue, heart, gastrointestinal tract, muscle, ligaments, and skin.
(2) Secondary amyloid, associated with chronic infections and rheumatoid arthritis, affecting liver, spleen, kidney, and adrenal.

A mixed pattern of (1) and (2) may occur in approximately 30 per cent of cases.

Clinical manifestations of primary amyloid are cardiac, gastro-intestinal with malabsorption, bleeding and diarrhoea, neuropathies, skin involvement with subcutaneous haemorrhage and purpura, macroglossia, xerostomia, and dysphagia.

Clinical manifestations of secondary amyloid are hepatosplenomegaly, renal and hepatic impairment, oedema, and nephrotic syndrome.

Dental Significance

The enlarged tongue is firm and shows indentations on the edges where it rests against the teeth. Mobility is reduced, which may result in speech impairment and poor oral hygiene. Patients should be instructed to clean their teeth efficiently after each meal as the tongue is unable to assist in this function.

Orthostatic hypotension is a common symptom and dentists who work on supine patients should elevate them from the horizontal slowly.

ANAEMIA

This is defined as a reduction in the concentration of haemoglobin in the peripheral blood below the normal, 13.5 g/100 ml in men, 11.5 g/100 ml in women. Anaemia may result from:

(1) blood loss;
(2) impaired red blood cell formation;
(3) increased red blood cell destruction.

The main types in these groups will be described.

(1) IRON DEFICIENCY ANAEMIA

This is the commonest type of anaemia. It occurs in all ages but most commonly in women of childbearing age. The major causes are excessive menstrual blood loss, gastrointestinal haemorrhage, and occasionally deficient diet or impaired iron absorption.

Besides general tiredness, nails may become brittle and spoon-shaped, papillae on the tongue atrophy, resulting in a smooth pale tongue, which may become red and sore. Rarely leukoplakia of the tongue occurs. Angular stomatitis with soreness and cracking at the angle of the mouth is common. A syndrome of iron deficiency anaemia, dysphagia, and glossitis (the Plummer–Vinson syndrome) is seen in middle-aged women, the dysphagia, resulting from a fine web in the post-cricoid region of the oesophagus. It is important to establish the cause of the anaemia to exclude serious underlying gastrointestinal disease. Treatment involves management of the underlying cause and iron supplements, usually oral, occasionally parenteral. Transfusion may be necessary where the anaemia is severe.

Dental Significance

Iron deficiency anaemia is common and is probably present in a tenth of the female population. The oral manifestations (atrophic glossitis, angular stomatitis, and sometimes aphthous ulceration) may be the presenting symptoms. When seen, the dentist should be alert to the likely underlying pathology, which can be confirmed by a blood picture.

Treatment is by oral **ferrous sulphate** or **ferrous fumarate** (*Fersamal*$_{GB}$, *Ferancee*$_{US}$), 200 mg three times daily after meals, and the patient's doctor should be informed so he can check there is no hidden cause of the anaemia. There are no contra-indications to routine dentistry, but treatment of the anaemia should be instituted before planning multiple extractions or oral surgery.

The oxygen-carrying capacity of the blood is reduced by the condition, and general anaesthetics should be conducted with a high concentration of oxygen in the anaesthetic gases to guard against cerebral anoxia. With haemoglobin levels below 10g/100ml. general anaesthesia should be postponed.

(2) MEGALOBLASTIC ANAEMIAS

These constitute 5 per cent of all anaemia and are caused by lack of vitamin B12, folate or both. The name derives from the appearance of the bone marrow.

Vitamin B12 deficiency gives rise to the following clinical manifestations:

(1) megaloblastic anaemia;
(2) glossitis;
(3) peripheral neuritis and subacute combined degeneration of the spinal cord.

The causes are:

(1) dietary deficiency, rare in this country except in strict vegetarians;
(2) intestinal disorders:
    (a) Addisonian pernicious anaemia results from a failure of the gastric antrum to produce intrinsic factor, which is essential for ileal absorption of B12;
    (b) bacterial contamination of the gut interfering with vitamin B12 absorption;
    (c) ileal disease (e.g. Crohn's);
    (d) surgical resection of the ileum.

A blood picture will reveal fewer red blood cells which are larger and contain full amounts of haemoglobin giving rise to the typical macrocytic normochromic anaemia with an increased MCV and normal MCHC. The white blood count and platelet count are frequently low and the polymorphonuclear cells show hypersegmentation of the nucleus.

It is of the utmost importance to establish the diagnosis before neurological complications occur as these may be irreversible. Treatment is with monthly injections of **hydroxocobalamin** (*Neocytamen*$_{GB}$) 1000 mg indefinitely. Care must be taken not to inadvertently treat B12 deficiency with folate as this may accelerate the neurological complications.

Folate deficiency results from inadequate intake, malabsorption, or increased demands such as in pregnancy and hypercatabolic states.

Clinical features are those of anaemia and glossitis. Treatment is with oral **folate** 5 mg BD until the underlying cause of the anaemia has been corrected.

Dental Significance

In all megaloblastic anaemias, whether of vitamin B12 or folate deficiency, atrophic glossitis, angular stomatitis, and mouth ulcers are common and may be the presenting symptoms of the condition. The dentist should be alert to the possibility when seeing patients with these signs in the mouth. The oral manifestations of the condition clear up quickly with correction of the deficiency.

NORMOCHROMIC NORMOCYTIC ANAEMIAS

These anaemias are not due to any deficiency but are the result of associated disease and respond only to correction of the causative disorder. They are seen in the following conditions:

(1) chronic infection, e.g. TB;
(2) renal failure;
(3) malignancy;
(4) liver disease;
(5) collagen disorders;
(6) endocrine disorders, e.g. myxoedema.

APLASTIC ANAEMIA

Aplasia of the bone marrow may be primary where the cause is unknown, or secondary to the toxic action of drugs, chemicals, and physical agents. Clinical features are those of the anaemia, such as tiredness, increased susceptibility to infection due to the leucopenia, and bleeding resulting from thrombocytopenia. It is commonly fatal, factors influencing prognosis are the aetiology, bleeding problems, and infection.

Dental Significance

Extensive oral ulceration and haemorrhagic gingivitis may be seen in the mouth as a result of the leucopenia. Extractions should be avoided and only carried out under antibiotic cover, anticipating increased post-extraction haemorrhage. Advice and assistance with oral hygiene is of paramount importance and local analgesics prescribed to ease discomfort (see LEUKAEMIA).

(3) HAEMOLYTIC ANAEMIAS

These result from increased breakdown of red blood cells occurring for the following reasons:

- Corpuscular defects
  - Hereditary spherocytosis
  - Hereditary haemaglobinopathies
    - thalassaemia
    - sickle cell disease

HEREDITARY SPHEROCYTOSIS

A defect in the red cell leads to its spherocytic shape. It is inherited as a Mendelian dominant, presenting with anaemia or jaundice. Complications include pigment gall stones, leg ulcers, splenomegaly, splenic infarction, and haemolytic crises. Diagnosis depends on the clinical and haematological features together with the family history. Treatment is by splenectomy.

THALASSAEMIAS

These are a group of inherited disorders due to defective synthesis of the α and β chains of haemoglobin.

β Thalassaemia major presents early in life with anaemia and splenomegaly, and in its severe form death often occurs in the first year of life. Milder forms are compatible with survival to adulthood.

β Thalassaemia minor (trait), the heterozygous form, is often symptomless, anaemia is mild and slight splenomegaly occurs. Life expectancy is normal. There is no specific treatment. Occasionally splenectomy is indicated and transfusion necessary.

α Thalassaemia major causes death of the foetus.

α Thalassaemia minor, the heterozygous form, is symptomless (high incidence in patients from Cyprus, Greece, and northern Italy).

SICKLE CELL DISEASE

In this hereditary disorder the red cells contain HbS, which is less soluble especially in its reduced form leading to deformity of the red cell and the characteristic sickle shape. It occurs most commonly in Negroes of African origin but is seen rarely in certain parts of southern Europe.

Clinical features result from chronic haemolytic anaemia and vascular obstruction due to high viscosity which results in ischaemia and infarction. Sickling crises occur, causing severe pain in bone, joints, and sometimes abdominal pain with vomiting. Gall stones are common. Central nervous system manifestations result from obstruction of cerebral vessels. Due to repeated splenic infarction the spleen is usually small in adults. Crises are precipitated by infection, stress, exposure to cold, fatigue, and anoxia. There is no specific treatment.

Dental Significance

Osteomyelitis of the mandible has been reported in those suffering from this condition but the main concern of the dentist lies in a sickling crisis being precipitated by anoxia under a general anaesthetic. The sickling trait can be detected by laboratory examination of the blood or by the dentist in the surgery using a Sickledex. Under ideal conditions all patients of West Indian or African origin should be tested before receiving a general anaesthetic, and, if positive, the anaesthetic administered in hospital. In areas with a large immigrant population this may present practical difficulties. Sickling only occurs with anoxia, and dental anaesthetics are not a hazard if this is remembered and the anaesthetic conducted with 50 per cent oxygen in the anaesthetic gases.

ACQUIRED HAEMOLYTIC ANAEMIA

This may be acute or chronic, idiopathic or secondary to a variety of causes, virus infection, drugs, underlying disease such as chronic lymphatic leukaemia, lymphomas, and systemic lupus erythematosus. It may occur at any age and in 50 per cent of cases is idiopathic.

Acute acquired haemolytic anaemia occurs most commonly in children and runs a short course usually with complete remission.

Chronic acquired haemolytic anaemia occurs mostly in adults and lasts months or years. It is usually associated with antibodies in the blood and is much commoner than the acute form.

Treatment consists of steroids, blood transfusion, and sometimes splenectomy. In most cases steroids will induce a remission.

Dental Significance

There are no contra-indications to routine dentistry but general anaesthetics should be conducted with a high concentration of oxygen in the anaesthetic gases and with special precautions if steroids have been used in treatment (see ADRENAL INSUFFICIENCY).

ANAPHYLAXIS

This is a type I, immediate hypersensitivity reaction in which the allergic agents combined to a protein component interact with IgE antibodies leading to a massive release of vasoactive compounds causing widespread vasodilatation and smooth muscle contraction. Most commonly it is the result of a drug reaction, usually following injection of the drug but it can occur after oral administration. The risk is greatly enhanced where there has been a previous reaction, often quite mild, such as a maculopapular rash. Initial symptoms are often a generalized pruritus, especially on the soles and palms, hyperaemia of the skin, angio-oedema, resulting in a fall in circulating blood volume, vascular collapse, and shock. The patient may experience a metallic taste in the mouth, an urge to micturate or defaecate and sometimes severe bronchospasm. Prolonged unconsciousness or vomiting may occur. Death may result from cardiac arrhythmias or asphyxia.

Prompt treatment is of paramount importance if lives are to be saved. Firstly clear the airway, if the patient has vomited, and administer oxygen. **Adrenaline** 0.5–1.0 ml of 1 in 1000 should be given intramuscularly and repeated at intervals of 5 minutes, if necessary, to sustain a measurable blood pressure. Subcutaneous adrenaline may not be absorbed fast enough and this route is not advised. In addition **hydrocortisone** 200 mg intravenously and an antihistamine such as **chlorpheniramine** 10 mg (*Piriton injection*$_{GB}$) intramuscularly should be given. As soon as resuscitation measures have been commenced arrangements should be made to transfer the patient to hospital with a dental or medical escort to continue treatment as required. An intravenous line should be established as soon as possible.

Dental Significance

Fortunately acute anaphylaxis is a rare sequel of drugs used in the dental surgery. Those more likely to provoke it are **penicillin, barbiturates** and anaesthetic agents. Brief questioning of the patient as to any previous experience is a wise precaution before using these.

ANEURISM, see VASCULAR DISEASE.

ANGINA PECTORIS, see HEART DISEASE (Ischaemic).

ANGIONEUROTIC OEDEMA

In the more common, non-hereditary form of this disease, swelling of the face and mouth can occur as an allergic reaction, though the particular allergen cannot always be traced. The oedema is not dangerous and subsides on its own in a number of days. Antihistamines, such as **chlorpheniramine** (Piriton$_{GB}$), 4 mg four times daily may help. A rare familial form of the disease results from an abnormality of the serum complement system. The oedema, which may involve the glottis, is sometimes provoked by trauma such as dental extractions. Prophylaxis with androgens and antifibrinolytic drugs has proved helpful in those subject to the condition. Treatment of an attack may require intramuscular **adrenaline** (0.5–1 ml of 1 in 1000),

hydrocortisone IV 100 mg, and tracheostomy if the airway is threatened.

Dental Significance

In the non-hereditary angioneurotic oedema the dentist should diligently enquire whether the attack appears to follow dental treatment, the fitting of any appliance, or the use of medicaments in the mouth. If so these should be avoided in the future.

Patients suffering from the familial form of the disease will usually be aware of it. Extractions and endodontics should be undertaken in hospital after infusion with fresh plasma.

ANKYLOSING SPONDYLITIS

This is an erosive inflammatory arthropathy affecting the sacroiliac joints and spine with a strong tendency to fixation of the spine. Most commonly it affects young men. There is a familial incidence and a characteristic tissue type HLA 27, indicating a genetic factor. Ulcerative colitis and Crohn's disease are seen more commonly with this condition than in the general population.

Dental Significance

Reclining dental chairs have made it easier to treat these patients in the surgery.

Occasionally the temporomandibular joint is involved in the disease and patients are unable to open their mouth more than 0.5 cm. Dental treatment must be adapted to what is possible with the limited access, and the patient helped with advice and mechanical aids to oral hygiene. General anaesthetics are a hazard and should only be administered in hospital.

ANOREXIA NERVOSA

This is a prolonged illness principally of young girls after puberty, characterized by gross weight loss which is self-induced, amenorrhoea, and psychological disturbance. The aetiology is unknown. Diagnosis is based on recognizing the clinical features of the illness and excluding organic disease, severe depressive illness, or schizophrenia. As the condition progresses hypotension, bradycardia, blue cold peripheries, and fine downy hair (lanugo) develop. Physical over-activity is often marked despite severe emaciation. There is no specific treatment but general management is of the greatest importance, the main aim – being the correction of the nutritional state and the psychiatric disturbance.

Dental Significance

Extensive enamel erosion is encountered either as a result of taking acid fruit juice or from purposeful vomiting after eating. It is most noticeable on the palatal surface of the upper incisors.

APLASTIC ANAEMIA, see ANAEMIA.

ASTHMA

This is a condition of variable breathlessness due to widespread narrowing of peripheral airways which varies in severity over short periods of time, spontaneously or with treatment. The narrowing results from release of various bronchoconstrictor substances in the bronchial wall. Many factors may influence their release: exercise, allergy, and infection. Psychological factors and drugs, especially beta-adrenergic blockers, may potentiate the effect. Asthma may be divided into:

(1) extrinsic asthma, occurring at a young age with a familial history of allergy, often in atopic subjects, running an intermittent course, associated with raised IgE levels;
(2) intrinsic asthma, occurring in middle age, usually persistent, associated with a family history of asthma, low levels of IgE, and unassociated with atopy.

Treatment

Where possible the allergen is eliminated. Desensitization may be possible. Drug therapy is aimed:

(a) to treat the acute attack;
(b) as a prophylactic measure to prevent attacks.

Treatment of Acute Attack

Sympathomimetic aerosols, **salbutamol** (*Ventolin*$_{GB}$), **terbutaline** (*Bricanyl*$_{GB}$, *Brethine*$_{US}$) or **orciprenaline** (*Alupent*$_{GB,US}$) are selective, and have a greater effect on the bronchi than the heart.

Prophylactic Treatment

Sodium cromoglycate (*Intal*$_{GB,US}$) spinhalers or steroid aerosols (**beclamethasone**) are most commonly used for prophylactic treatment. Theophylline derivatives (**aminophylline**) and cholinergic drugs are also of value.

TREATMENT OF A SEVERE ATTACK

Put a face mask on the patient and give oxygen. Next, 200 mg of **hydrocortisone** should be given intravenously followed by the slow intravenous injection of 250 mg **aminophylline** in 10 ml of water, given at the rate of 1 ml (25 mg) per minute. Arrangements should be made to transfer the patient to hospital as soon as possible.

Dental Significance

There are no contra-indications to routine dentistry with local anaesthetics but patients should be instructed to take the prophylactic measures they have been prescribed and bring with them any aerosol that they use in an attack.

General anaesthetics may be given to those who suffer from mild uncomplicated asthma providing certain precautions are taken. If possible a time of the year should be chosen where attacks are less frequent. Normal prophylactic treatment should be taken and aerosols brought with the patient. **Atropine** should be given as a premedication (0.2 mg under 10 years, 0.4–0.6 mg over 10 years and adults) either intramuscularly 1 hour before or intravenously at the time of the anaesthetic. If intravenous induction is desired, the amount should be no more than that required to put the patient to sleep and then anaesthesia induced and maintained with 50 per cent oxygen, nitrous oxide, and halothane to concentration required. The drugs required to treat a severe attack of asthma should be readily available.

ATHEROMA, see VASCULAR DISEASE.

AURICULAR FIBRILLATION, see HEART DISEASE (DYSRHYTHMIC).

B

B

BACTERIAL ENDOCARDITIS, see **HEART DISEASE (Infective), SUBACUTE BACTERIAL ENDOCARDITIS**

BEHÇET'S SYNDROME

This condition, seen more frequently in the Mediterranean countries and Japan is of unknown aetiology. Painful aphthous-type ulcers occur in the mouth and on the genitals together with conjunctivitis or iridocyclitis. A skin eruption, recurrent arthritis affecting arms and legs, and neurological signs may be present. Systemic corticosteroids and immuno-suppressive drugs are used to combat the condition but, unlike Reiter's disease which it resembles, Behçet's syndrome tends to be chronic and poorly influenced by treatment.

Dental Significance

Triamcinolone paste (*Adcortyl*$_{\text{GB}}$, *Kenalog*$_{\text{US}}$) in orobase, or **betamethasone** spray (*Betnesol*$_{\text{GB}}$) to the mouth ulcers four times daily is usually helpful.

BELL'S PALSY

This unilateral facial paralysis is probably due to localized neuritis of the 7th nerve within the bony canal, the cause of which is unknown. It affects both sexes equally and can occur at any age. The onset is sudden, a patient usually complaining of stiffness in the face when getting up in the morning, and paralysis developing over the next 24–48 hours. Bilateral and recurrent palsy are occasionally encountered, and there is a similar condition (Ramsay Hunt syndrome) which is due to herpes zoster of the geniculate ganglion and where the facial paralysis is accompanied by vesicles round the ear. Recovery starts after a week but the prognosis is less favourable in the old and in those in whom the paralysis is total.

Steroids, given as soon as possible after diagnosis, offer the best chance of reducing nerve damage. **Prednisolone**, 20 mg four times a day, should be given for 5 days and then the dosage tailed off over another 3 days.

Dental Significance

Because of the disfigurement and embarrassment of facial paralysis, a dentist seeing a patient with the early symptoms of Bell's palsy should contact the patient's doctor and, with his blessing, commence treatment with steroids immediately; providing the patient does not suffer from diabetes mellitus or peptic ulceration.

In those with severe paralysis an acrylic-covered wire hook, set in a part upper denture, may be helpful in holding up the corner of the mouth to prevent dribbling. Food often accumulates in the buccal sulcus and instruction and assistance in oral hygiene is important.

BILIARY DISEASE

CHOLANGITIS

Infection of the extrahepatic or intrahepatic biliary tree usually complicates obstruction of the bile ducts due to gallstones, surgery, or other causes. The clinical picture is of an acute, often severe, illness characterized by abdominal pain, jaundice, fever, and rigors.

Treatment requires high doses of systemic antibiotics but in the case of biliary obstruction surgical correction of the obstruction may be necessary to control the infection.

CHOLECYSTITIS

Inflammation of the gall bladder is frequently, but not always, associated with gallstones. Acute cholecystitis causes abdominal pain, usually over the gall bladder area, tenderness, and fever. It is most common in middle-aged women. Complications include perforation, empyema, and gangrene of the gall bladder. Treatment is conservative with antibiotics and, provided the patient is responding, with elective surgery at a later date. If the patient is deteriorating urgent surgery may be indicated. Chronic cholecystitis is a poorly understood entity. Flatulent dyspepsia and vague upper abdominal pains are frequently attributed to it, but there is no doubt these symptoms are common in people with normal gall bladders, and cholecystectomy frequently fails to cure the symptoms.

GALLSTONES

Gallstones result from a disorder of bile secretion in the liver but the stones usually form in the gall bladder rather than the bile ducts. Seventy to eighty per cent of gallstones are asymptomatic. They occur more commonly in women than men, particularly in those who have had children and frequency increases with age. Forty to seventy per cent of women have gallstones by the time they reach old age.

Most gallstones are predominantly cholesterol. Pigment gallstones are seen particularly in the presence of haemolytic blood disorders. The clinical features result from the gallstones obstructing the neck of the gall bladder or common bile duct. The pain is often severe, persistent, and frequently related to eating, especially fatty food. An obstructing stone in the gall bladder, which does not pass spontaneously, results in either cholecystitis or a (symptomless) non-functioning gall bladder. Obstruction to the common bile duct causes jaundice, sometimes associated with ascending cholangitis and pancreatitis.

Treatment for symptomatic gall stones is surgical. However, under certain circumstances—for example, where there are strong contra-indications to surgery and where the gallstones are radiolucent—dissolution of the gallstones, using **chenodeoxycholic acid** (*Chendol*$_{GB}$) or **ursodeoxycholic acid** (*Destolit*$_{GB}$) is sometimes successful.

Dental Significance

Jaundice, when present, will be evident in the mucous membrane of the mouth as well as the skin and sclerae of the eyes. With obstructive jaundice there is malabsorption of vitamin K and intramuscular fat-soluble vitamin K, **menadiol sodium phosphate** 10 mg (*Synkavit*$_{GB}$, *Synkayvite*$_{US}$) should be given 8 hours prior to any dental extraction.

General anaesthetics should be administered in hospital, and halothane avoided as an anaesthetic agent.

BORNHOLM'S DISEASE (epidemic myalgia, pleurodynia)

This condition is caused by Coxsackie virus of the B group. The incubation period is 2–14 days and symptoms develop suddenly with headache, fever, and severe pain in the lower chest, abdomen, and sometimes limbs. The acute phase usually passes in 2–3 days but fever and less severe pains may last for a week. There is no specific treatment and the prognosis is good.

Dental Significance

None.

BRONCHIECTASIS

In this condition there is irreversible dilatation of the bronchi, most commonly secondary to infection and obstruction. It usually develops in childhood. It may be localized or widespread and bilateral. Symptoms are of a cough productive of large volumes of purulent sputum. Often the patient remains well with little incapacity. Physical signs include finger clubbing and coarse creps in the areas affected. Haemoptysis is a common feature. Complications include pneumonia and rarely pericarditis, cerebral abscess, and amyloid.

Treatment consists of teaching the patient effective postural drainage and the use of antibiotics, either in exacerbations of the disease or on a long-term basis. For localized disease surgery may be successful. Prognosis in general is good.

Dental Significance

None, unless associated with impaired ventilatory capacity (see BRONCHITIS), or secondary amyloid (see AMYLOIDOSIS).

BRONCHITIS (chronic)

The symptoms of chronic bronchitis result from excessive production of bronchial secretions giving rise to a productive cough on most days for at least 3 months in the year. Because it is frequently associated with airway obstruction variable degrees of emphysema are common. Chronic bronchitis is closely associated with smoking, working in dusty conditions, poor social circumstances, and an urban environment. Initial symptoms consist only of a productive cough but as the condition progresses increasing dyspnoea occurs, leading to progressive respiratory failure. In a proportion of patients right-sided heart failure occurs (cor pulmonale).

Management—Patients who smoke should stop, and where possible avoid dusty environments. Antibiotics should be used for exacerbations but not on a long-term basis. Where there is significant airway obstruction, bronchodilators should be used and in the more resistant patients steroids may be very beneficial. Complications include pneumonia, pneumothorax, polycythaemia, cor pulmonale, and respiratory failure.

Dental Significance

General anaesthetics in patients suffering from chronic bronchitis are a hazard. Many bronchitics exist with a raised level of carbon dioxide in the blood and reduced oxygen tension. When this is altered through breathing anaesthetic gases containing higher levels of oxygen and no carbon dioxide, stimulation to breathe ceases. Any patient whose bronchitis is such as to require medical treatment should be referred for an anaesthetic assessment before a general anaesthetic is administered.

BRUCELLOSIS (undulant fever)

This is primarily an animal disease, with man becoming an accidental host, either through contact with infected animals or by consumption of infected milk, cream or cheese.

The disease is caused by the bacteria *Brucella*, of which there are three species: *B. abortus* mainly in cattle, *B. melitensis* in goat and sheep, and *B. suis* in swine. *Brucella* can invade via the gastrointestinal tract, skin, respiratory tract, or conjunctiva. The incubation period may be from 2 weeks to many months. The disease may be acute with rigors, sweats, fever, headache, and depression. However, the severity of symptoms varies and the illness may be no more than a mild 'flu-like illness.

In the chronic form there may be no acute phase and symptoms include depression, headaches, weakness, sweating, backache, anorexia, and insomnia. Diagnosis is confirmed by culturing the organism from a blood sample in the acute phase of the illness, or serological tests.

Treatment in the acute phase is very effective, **tetracycline** (250–500 mg 6-hourly) being the drug of choice. In the chronic form treatment may have little or no effect.

Dental Significance

Stomatitis, with numerous small ulcers and oedematous gingivae, has been reported but is not common.

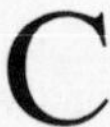

CANDIDA INFECTION (Thrush)

Infection with the fungus *Candida albicans* can be localized to the mouth, may be acute or chronic or spread widely over the body. The severe form, characterized by large white patches on the tongue, buccal mucosa, and elsewhere, is usually associated with immunodeficiency disease, debility, diabetes, malignancy, or prolonged treatment with antibiotics, corticosteroids, or cytotoxic drugs. A chronic atrophic form is seen under upper dentures and orthodontic appliances.

Chronic mucocutaneous candidiasis is always associated with an immunological defect and is seen in different forms in the young and elderly.

Treatment must be aimed firstly at correcting the predisposing factors, general or local. Severe infections require systemic treatment, but if mild and localized to the mouth, topical applications of fungicides held in the mouth for several minutes four times daily will be effective. Preparations include **nystatin** (*Nystatin*$_{GB}$ mixture) (*Mycostatin*$_{US}$ oral suspension), **amphotericin** lozenges (*Fungilin*$_{GB}$), **miconazole** (*Daktarin*$_{GB}$), and **ketoconazole.** Infection of the skin should be treated with 1 per cent **clotrimazole** cream, (*Canesten*$_{GB}$) (*Mycelex*$_{US}$, *Lotrimin*$_{US}$).

Dental Significance

The diagnosis of acute oral thrush is usually obvious but can be confirmed by scraping off one of the white patches which will show the typical hyphae when examined microscopically. The chronic form seen under an appliance must be distinguished from allergy to the appliance material. The denture or appliance should be left out at night, and it is usually advised that it be left soaking in 0.2 per cent **chlorhexidine** solution and coated with a fungicidal gel (*Nystangel*$_{GB}$), (*Mycostatin*$_{US}$ oral suspension) before reinsertion. However recent research has thrown doubt on the value of the latter.

C

Candida leukoplakia appearing in the floor of the mouth or on the sides of the tongue must be considered as precancerous (see LEUKOPLAKIA).

CARCINOID SYNDROME

This condition is characterized by flushing, diarrhoea, wheezing, and cardiac disease and is due to secretion of various vasoactive substances, 5-hydroxytryptamine, bradykinin, and histamine by carcinoid tumour tissue. These tumours arise from the argentaffin cells of the gut and are most frequently found in the ileum. The syndrome only occurs once the tumour has metastasized to the liver, and thus the prognosis for the syndrome is usually poor. The most common symptom is flushing which is paroxysmal but may be precipitated by certain foods, alcohol, and excitement. Diarrhoea is variable and not always present. Like the flushing, asthma is paroxysmal and usually accompanies the flushing when present. In carcinoid heart disease the right side of the heart is more commonly affected. Fibrous tissue is laid down on the endothelium of the heart causing pulmonary stenosis and tricuspid incompetence. Diagnosis is confirmed by measuring the metabolite 5-hydroxyindolacetic acid in the urine. Treatment is mainly symptomatic; rarely is surgery indicated or of benefit.

Dental Significance

As stated, the prognosis in this condition is poor though patients may survive for several years. Dentistry must be planned with this in mind. By reason of the cardiac and bronchial complication, general anaesthetics should be avoided, and if essential administered in hospital.

CARDIAC ARREST, see HEART DISEASE (Ischaemic).

CHICKEN POX, see VARICELLA.

CHOLANGITIS, see BILIARY DISEASE.

CHOLECYSTITIS, see BILIARY DISEASE.

CHOREA

HUNTINGTON'S CHOREA

This disease is inherited as a Mendelian dominant, although sporadic cases occur. It appears between the ages of 30 and 45 and progresses from choreiform movements to dementia and complete incapacity. The duration of the disease is 5–30 years. The cause is unknown. There is no treatment other than sedation.

Dental Significance

If dental procedures have to be performed a general anaesthetic will be necessary, because only then will the athetoid movements cease.

SYDENHAM'S CHOREA (St. Vitus' dance)

This is a condition characterized by complex involuntary movements which are variable and may involve several muscles. The cause is unknown but is thought to be rheumatic inflammation of the brain in view of its association with acute rheumatism and rheumatic heart disease. It is now rare but was common 25 years ago. It occurs between the ages of 5 and 15, often associated with emotional instability. Recovery occurs in 6 weeks to 3 months.

Treatment is by complete bed rest and careful nursing. **Salicylates** are of value and sedation may be beneficial.

Dental Significance

A medical history of Sydenham's chorea will alert the dentist to the likelihood of valvular disease of the heart. Antibiotic cover will be required for dental procedures likely to cause a bacteraemia (see HEART DISEASE (infective). SUBACUTE BACTERIAL ENDOCARDITIS). General anaesthetics should not be given without an assessment by a physician.

CHRISTMAS DISEASE, see HAEMOPHILIA.

CIRRHOSIS, see LIVER DISEASE.

COARCTATION OF THE AORTA, see HEART DISEASE (Congenital).

COELIAC DISEASE

One in two thousand of the general population suffers with coeliac disease in the United Kingdom, and it constitutes the commonest cause of malabsorption. More than one member of a family may have the condition which is associated with the skin condition, dermatitis herpetiformis and the tissue type HLAB8. The basic defect is due to a poorly understood interaction between a fraction of gluten (alphagliaden) and the small intestinal mucosa. This results in damage and flattening of the mucosal villi. The clinical consequences of this 'flat' mucosa are diarrhoea and weight loss together with other features of malabsorption such as anaemia and osteomalacia. Mouth ulceration is an unexplained associated finding. The condition may present in infancy with diarrhoea and failure to thrive, or for the first time in adult life. Diarrhoea may be absent, making diagnosis difficult and delayed.

Once suspected the diagnosis is confirmed with a jejunal biopsy and by observing improvement on a gluten-free diet. Such a diet leads to complete recovery; however gluten is contained in all cereal crops, and all food products made from them have to be constituted from specially prepared flour.

Untreated, the disease may lead to severe malnutrition and death, a serious but rare complication being small bowel lymphoma.

Dental Significance

Recurrent aphthous ulcers are seen in about a quarter of patients with this disease. They clear up with treatment of the primary condition but resolution may be assisted by topical steroids in the form of **hydrocortisone** lozenges 2.5 mg (*Corlan*$_{GB}$) or *triamcinolone* paste (*Adcortyl*$_{GB}$, *Kenalog*$_{US}$) in orobase.

Enamel hypoplasia is found when the disease has been present since infancy and the signs of osteomalacia when it has remained untreated.

Anaemia is a common complication and must be borne in mind if general anaesthetics are required.

COLITIS

The term means inflammation of the colon. The main causes are given below.

(1) SPECIFIC COLITIS

pseudomembranous colitis
ischaemic colitis
radiation colitis
infective colitis
  amoebic
  tuberculous

(2) NON-SPECIFIC COLITIS

ulcerative colitis
Crohn's colitis.

PSEUDOMEMBRANOUS COLITIS

This condition presents with typical colitic symptoms, rectal bleeding, diarrhoea, and abdominal pain. It is most commonly the result of antibiotics, particularly **clindamycin** (*Dalacin C*$_{GB}$, *Cleocin*$_{US}$) and **lincomycin** (*Lincocin*$_{GB,US}$) although it has now been reported following almost all antibiotics. It results from the effects of a toxin produced by the bacterium *Clostridium deficile*. This can be isolated from the stools and the toxin can be identified. In the florid form of the disease the large bowel mucosa has a characteristic appearance, being partly covered by white plaques which when removed leave a bleeding area of mucosa. The condition can vary from a mild diarrhoeal illness to severe total colitis, sometimes requiring colectomy. There is unfortunately no way of predicting who is liable to develop this complication of antibiotic therapy, and the worrying fact is that it can develop following only very limited courses of antibiotics.

Treatment is symptomatic. Specific treatment is with **vamcamycin** or **metronidazole.**

ISCHAEMIC COLITIS

This condition is most commonly seen in the elderly and results from arteriosclerotic disease of the mesenteric vessels. It may present acutely with bloody diarrhoea which may progress to gut infarction, or it may present with diarrhoea associated with ischaemic stricture formation. Treatment is symptomatic.

ULCERATIVE COLITIS

This inflammatory disease of the colon is of unknown aetiology and more common in the second to fourth decades. In the west its prevalence is 5 per 100,000. The severity of the condition varies from a mild intermittent diarrhoeal illness to a life-threatening disease. The direct complications include toxic dilation of the colon, perforation, massive bleeding and carcinoma, while indirect complications are uveitis, iritis, erythema nodosum, arthritis, and cirrhosis.

Treatment consists of symptomatic treatment of the diarrhoea with **codeine phosphate, diphenoxylate** (*Lomotil*$_{\mathrm{GB}}$), or **loperamide hydrochloride** (*Imodium*$_{\mathrm{GB,US}}$) and anti-inflammatory treatment with **sulphasalazine** (*Salazopyrin*$_{\mathrm{GB}}$, *Azulfidine*$_{\mathrm{US}}$) and **prednisolone** given either systemically or topically in the form of enemas or suppositories. Surgery (colectomy) is curative but almost invariably results in a permanent ileostomy.

Dental Significance

Recurrent aphthous ulceration of the mouth is not uncommon in patients with ulcerative colitis. Its severity corresponds to that of the bowel condition and improves with medical or surgical treatment of the primary disease. Topical steroids in the form of **hydrocortisone** pellets (*Corlan*$_{GB}$) or **triamcinolone** paste (*Adcortyl*$_{GB}$), (*Kenalog*$_{US}$) in orobase, are helpful. If discomfort is severe a viscous mouthwash containing 2 per cent **lignocaine** will make eating less of a misery. Dentists must appreciate that most cases of pseudomembranous colitis are the direct result of treatment with antibiotics, especially **clindamycin** (*Dalacin C*$_{GB}$, *Cleocin*$_{US}$) and **lincomycin** (*Lincocin*$_{GB,US}$). No antibiotic should be prescribed without good cause, and these two only for infections where the organism is insensitive to safer alternatives.

Patients under treatment with **diphenoxylate** and **atropine** (*Lomotil*$_{GB}$) may suffer from xerostomia and conscientious attention to oral hygiene and caries control is most important. Those receiving **prednisolone** systemically or rectally must be treated as cases of adrenal insufficiency and appropriate precautions taken (see ADRENAL INSUFFICIENCY).

CONN'S SYNDROME, see ADRENAL DISEASE.

CORONARY THROMBOSIS, see HEART DISEASE (Ischaemic).

COR PULMONALE

This is a right-sided heart failure secondary to obstruction in the pulmonary circulation or more commonly chronic lung disease.

Dental Significance

General anaesthetics are to be avoided.

CRANIAL ARTERITIS

This condition results from a granulomatous arteritis and is confined to the elderly. Severe headache and scalp tenderness are the cardinal features, though symptoms may be very similar to those of polymyalgia rheumatica. Occasionally fever and malaise are the only features. The all-important complication is rapid development of blindness, and as soon as the diagnosis is made urgent treatment with systemic steroids is mandatory. Diagnosis is confirmed by temporal artery biopsy.

Dental Significance

As in polymyalgia rheumatica, jaw-ache and tenderness of masseter and temporal muscles may be a prominent complaint. Dentists should enquire if corticosteroids have been taken in the last 3 months and act accordingly (see ADRENAL INSUFFICIENCY).

CRETINISM, see THYROID DISEASE.

CROHN'S DISEASE

This inflammatory bowel disease of unknown aetiology occurs most commonly between the second and fourth decade and appears to be increasing in incidence. Any part of the bowel may be affected from mouth to anus, the distribution being characteristically patchy and the full thickness of the bowel being involved.

Presentation is extremely variable, abdominal pain and diarrhoea being the commonest symptoms but anorexia, weight loss, fever, night sweats, vomiting, and anaemia may all occur as presenting features with or without diarrhoea.

Diagnosis is based on radiological and histological appearances.

In addition to symptomatic treatment for pain and diarrhoea, replacement therapy is required for nutritional deficiencies and specific anti-inflammatory treatment for control of the disease. The choice of drug is extremely limited. **Prednisolone** is the only generally effective medical treatment, the dose being varied between 5 and 60 mg/day depending on the severity of the disease. **Sulphasalazine** (*Salazopyrin*$_{GB}$, *Azulfidine*$_{US}$) (2–4 g/day) may be beneficial in colonic but not small bowel Crohn's disease. Immunosuppressive therapy is of no proven value.

Remissions and relapses are the pattern of the disease. There is no known cure. Surgery when necessary is conservative, in view of the recurrent nature of the disease. Complications are similar to those seen in ulcerative colitis.

Dental Significance

Oral ulceration, varying from mild aphthous to deep indurated ulcers, is seen in some 10 per cent of patients suffering from Crohn's disease. Areas of the mucous membrane of the mouth may show granulomatous infiltration similar to that found in the small intestine. Topical steroid treatment with **hydrocortisone** pellets (*Corlan*$_{GB}$) or **triamcinolone** paste (*Adcortyl*$_{GB}$, *Kenalog*$_{US}$) in orobase, is usually effective and **chlorhexidine** 0.2 per cent (*Corsodyl*$_{GB}$) as a mouthwash used four times a day will prevent secondary infection. If discomfort is severe a viscous mouthwash containing 2 per cent **lignocaine** will make eating less of a misery.

Anaemia and adrenal insufficiency (by reason of treatment with steroids) must be taken into account if general anaesthetics are required (see ADRENAL INSUFFICIENCY).

CUSHING'S DISEASE, see ADRENAL DISEASE.

CYSTIC FIBROSIS (fibrocystic disease, mucoviscidosis)

This condition is due to a defect of cell membrane function resulting in diminished sodium reabsorption. Body secretions are abnormal in either viscosity or volume. There are three main clinical manifestations of this inherited defect:

(1) Meconium ileus. The viscid mucus results in solidification of intestinal contents in the neonate with intestinal obstruction. The prognosis is extremely poor.
(2) Gastrointestinal. Chronic diarrhoea and steatorrhoea occur due to pancreatic insufficiency resulting from obstruction to pancreatic ducts by viscous secretions.
(3) Respiratory. Recurrent infections lead to bronchiectasis and emphysema. If untreated 80 per cent die in the first year of life, usually from bronchopneumonia. With prompt treatment of super-added infections 75 per cent may reach adolescence. However, mean survival in the best centres is only 12 years.

Dental Significance

Chronic sinusitis is a feature of the condition and enlargement of the submandibular salivary glands has been reported. General anaesthetics should only be administered in hospital.

D

D

DEMENTIA, see PSYCHIATRIC DISORDERS.

DERMATOMYOSITIS

This is a collagen disorder characterized by diffuse inflammation of skin and muscle, the cause of which is unknown. Women are affected twice as often as men, and the peak age is between 30 and 50. In 15 per cent of adults there is an associated underlying carcinoma.

The symptoms are malaise, myalgia, weakness, and fatigue. The rash occurs over the V of the neck and extensor surfaces of the limbs. Erythema can affect the face giving a typical heliotrope colour with periorbital oedema.

Diagnosis is clinical and may be confirmed by muscle biopsy.

Steroids are the mainstay of medical treatment. Surgery may be indicated for underlying malignancy and can lead to symptomatic improvement. In general prognosis is poor, 50 per cent of patients dying in 3 years.

Dental Significance

In a number of cases oedema of the mucous membranes and a red–blue erythema is found in the mouth. Steroid treatment must be taken into consideration if extractions are contemplated (see ADRENAL INSUFFICIENCY). General anaesthetics should be administered in hospital.

DIABETES INSIPIDUS

This condition results from deficient production of antidiuretic hormone due to disease or damage to the hypothalamus or posterior pituitary. The symptoms of polyuria and polydipsia may rapidly lead to severe dehydration if fluid losses cannot be replaced.

Treatment involves correction of the underlying cause where possible and replacement therapy with **antidiuretic hormone** (*Lypressin*$_{GB}$, *Pitressin*$_{US}$) administered as a nasal spray or in more severe cases as an intramuscular injection.

Dental Significance

None.

DIABETES MELLITUS

This is a clinical syndrome caused by the derangement of carbohydrate, fat, and protein metabolism resulting from a deficiency of insulin. It is common; 12–14 per cent of adults having an abnormal glucose tolerance curve. There are approximately 400,000 people with clinical diabetes in England and Wales at the present time.

The aetiology is not clear but there is an inherited tendency to diabetes and a close correlation with obesity.

Diabetes may be latent and brought on by stress, asymptomatic with abnormal biochemistry only or symptomatic. The majority of diabetics fall into one of two groups:

(1) *the juvenile type* in which those afflicted are typically young thin, ketotic, insulin-dependent, and the diabetes insulin-sensitive;

(2) *maturity-onset* in which the diabetics tend to be obese, non-ketotic, have mild symptoms, are often not insulin-dependent and the condition is insulin-resistant.

The clinical presentation may be very variable. The insulin-dependent diabetic may present acutely with the classical features of diabetic ketoacidosis, severe thirst, polyuria, loss of weight, vomiting, and anorexia. On examination the patient is dehydrated, over-breathing, drowsy, occasionally comatose, and with a smell of ketones on the breath. By contrast diabetes may be a chance finding complicating other diseases, or may present with the complications of the disease itself.

Diagnosis depends on the glucose tolerance test with a 2-hour blood glucose level greater than 160 mg/100 ml.

Being a multisystem disease complications can be multiple and varied. Vision may be impaired due to cataract formation and diabetic retinopathy. Renal function may be affected due either to the increased tendency to renal infection or to intrinsic renal damage leading to glomerulosclerosis and renal failure (Kimmelstiel–Wilson kidney). Infections generally are more common. Atherosclerosis involves both large and small arteries leading to an increased risk of cerebral and cardiovascular complications, and skin ulceration associated with small-vessel involvement. The nervous system can be affected either centrally or peripherally, giving rise to acute and chronic peripheral neuropathy, autonomic neuropathy, diabetic amyotrophy, neuropathic ulceration, impotence, and diarrhoea.

Treatment may be subdivided as follows:

(1) Diet alone. Obese elderly patients with no ketosis may be managed with a low-carbohydrate diet.

(2) Oral hypoglycaemic agents. In non-ketotic patients, where diet does not suffice to control the blood sugar, oral hypoglycaemic agents may be used. There are two types:

(a) Sulphonylureas

(i) **Tolbutamide** (*Rastinon*$_{GB}$, *Orinase*$_{US}$). A short-acting agent.

(ii) **Chlorpropamide** (*Diabinese*$_{GB,US}$). A long-acting agent.

(iii) **Glibenclamide** (*Daonil*$_{GB}$). An intermediate-acting agent.

These augment insulin secretion

(b) Biguanides

(i) **Metformin** (*Glucophage*$_{GB}$).

(ii) **Phenformin** (*Dibotin*$_{GB}$).

These inhibit glucose absorption from the gut and glucose oxidation.

(3) **Insulin.** Underweight patients with ketosis should always be treated with insulin, of which there are three main types: short-, intermediate-, and long-acting. Many highly purified insulins are now available reducing the tendency to allergic reactions and immunological resistance to insulin.

(4) Emergency treatment of diabetic ketosis and coma. Treatment of these emergency situations requires hospital admission. The main aspects of treatment are rehydration, administration of soluble **insulin**, correction of acid–base imbalance, and management of complications.

HYPOGLYCAEMIA AND HYPOGLYCAEMIC COMA

These result from excessive therapy with oral agents and insulin, or normal therapy in the presence of inadequate calorie intake.

Symptoms are hunger, faintness, sweating, and aggressiveness progressing to coma. Treatment is with oral **glucose** in the co-operative conscious patient and intravenous **dextrose** (50 ml of 50 per cent dextrose) in the presence of pre-coma or coma.

If treated, hypoglycaemic coma does not carry the serious consequences of hyperglycaemic coma and admission to hospital may not be necessary. Delay in treatment can lead to irreversible brain damage.

Dental Significance

Because oral manifestations may be among the first, the dentist often plays an important part in the diagnosis of this disease or in warning sufferers when blood sugar control is inadequate. Xerostomia, associated with a bad taste and a burning tongue, is a frequent complaint. *Candida* patches, paradontal disease, and an unexplained increase in caries are other features. Bell's palsy is more common in diabetics.

Scrupulous oral hygiene is important. Routine dental treatment requires no special precautions, but general anaesthetics must be approached with care. Those patients whose diabetes is adequately controlled by diet or oral hypoglycaemics, can be given general anaesthetics in the dental surgery but the morning dose of hypoglycaemic is best omitted to compensate for pre-anaesthetic fasting (hyperglycaemia is safer than hypoglycaemia). Patients who require **insulin** to control their condition should only receive general anaesthetics in hospital where their blood sugar can be monitored.

Aspirin can enhance the effect of oral hypoglycaemic agents, if taken in quantity. Alternative analgesics should be prescribed to relieve dental pain in diabetic patients being treated with these drugs.

HYPO- VERSUS HYPERGLYCAEMIC COMA

The dental practitioner may be worried about the distinction between hyper- and hypoglycaemic coma. In practice this problem is unlikely to arise and is not difficult to resolve if it does. Hyperglycaemic coma develops gradually in a patient who is clearly ill and unlikely to be visiting his dentist. As infection is the commonest precipitating factor, the patient is usually toxic and febrile with a hot dry skin and ketotic breath. Hypoglycaemia usually results from inappropriate **insulin** dosage and develops rapidly, usually in a patient who has been quite well up until the time of the coma. Prodromal symptoms are faintness, sweating, hunger, and aggressiveness. The comatose patient is not febrile or ketotic. If in doubt intravenous **glucose** therapy will rapidly resolve the problem, rousing the patient with hypoglycaemia and having no effect on the patient with hyperglycaemia who needs to be transferred urgently to hospital.

DIVERTICULAR DISEASE

This term is most commonly applied to the presence of diverticula in the colon. These are herniations of the mucous membrane through the muscle wall of the gut. They may occur throughout the colon but are usually found in the sigmoid region. The condition is extremely common in western society, 30 per cent of the population over 60 years of age being affected.

Symptoms consist of abdominal pain and alteration in bowel habit, but in the majority of cases the condition is symptomless.

Complications include bleeding, inflammation, and abscess formation (diverticulitis).

Dental Significance

None.

DIVERTICULITIS, see DIVERTICULAR DISEASE.

DOWN'S SYNDROME (Mongolism)

The condition results from chromosome imbalance and has a frequency of 1 in 650 live births. It is more common in children of older mothers.

There is mental deficiency of a variable degree and impaired resistance to infections. Cardiac and skeletal defects are not uncommon and the incidence of diabetes, hypothyroidism, and leukaemia increased. There is no treatment, but children brought up in the home overcome their difficulties better than those in institutions.

Dental Significance

A large fissured tongue, an open bite, and a Class III malocclusion are the usual presenting features. Delayed eruption with missing or malformed teeth is frequent. Liability to caries is not increased but periodontal disease and ulcerative gingivitis are common problems.

Generally, the children are co-operative and, with careful handling, routine dental treatment can be undertaken.

A mouth-gag may help a child to keep his mouth open and be a precaution against being bitten. Local anaesthetics should be used where required and sedation may be helpful, though unpredictable. The importance of oral hygiene should be stressed.

Antibiotic cover (**penicillin V** or **amoxycillin** 250 mg three times daily) is advised for extractions, while general anaesthetics should be approached with care because of the likelihood of cardiac abnormalities. Mongols cared for in institutions are more likely to be carriers of hepatitis B, and should be treated as high-risk cases in this respect.

DUODENAL ULCER, see PEPTIC ULCER.

DYSTROPHIA MYOTONICA

This is a hereditary disorder appearing between the ages of 20 and 30 and characterized by myotonia and muscle-wasting. The wasting is seen in the facial muscles, sternomastoids, shoulder girdle, forearms, quadriceps, and leg muscles. In addition cataracts, frontal balding, dementia, and in men gonadal atrophy and impotence occur. In women amenorhoea is usual.

Dental Significance

General anaesthetics should be avoided and, if essential, administered in hospital.

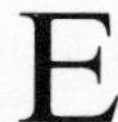

EATON-LAMBERT SYNDROME, see MYASTHENIC SYNDROME.

ECZEMA

Eczema is a reaction of the skin in response to some damaging stimulus which may not be identifiable. Atopic eczema is usually seen in young children, starting on the face and spreading to antecubital and popliteal areas. It is frequently associated with asthma. Subacute and chronic eczema may result from direct skin irritation with chemicals, detergents, cosmetics, or from allergy to drugs or topical medicaments. It is frequently influenced by psychological factors. Infection may complicate it.

Attempts should be made to discover and avoid the precipitating agent. Treatment includes the use of emollients, antimicrobials, antihistamines, and corticosteroids.

Dental Significance

If systemic **cortisone** has been used in the treatment of the condition, this must be taken into account if oral surgery or general anaesthetics are planned (see ADRENAL INSUFFICIENCY).

Dentists and their assistants should try and avoid unnecessary skin contact with medicaments and materials used in their profession.

EHLERS-DANLOS SYNDROME

This condition results from an abnormality of collagen in connective tissue. The skin and mucous membranes are more fragile than normal, and damage and haemorrhage occur with minimal trauma. The teeth are frequently deformed with stunted roots and multiple pulp-stones. Periodontal disease is common.

Dental Significance

A gentle touch is essential when working on these patients. Though there is no clotting defect, increased haemorrhage must be expected after extractions and sutures do not hold adequately in the gingiva. Dislocation of the temporomandibular joint has been reported.

EMBOLISM

This is the blockage of a blood vessel by a clot or collection of abnormal material within the vascular compartment, which has been carried to that site by the blood stream.

Fat emboli may complicate fractures and orthopaedic procedures.

Air emboli occur following trauma or surgical and medical procedures involving large vessels.

PULMONARY EMBOLI

By far the commonest type of embolus is a blood clot and the commonest sites of origin are the deep leg veins or pelvic veins. The clot embolizes to the lungs and may cause immediate fatal obstruction to the pulmonary arterial system. More commonly emboli present with pleuritic pain and haemoptysis. They are seen most commonly in ill, immobile people, and constitute a major postoperative complication. An association has been recognized between the contraceptive pill and pulmonary emboli in otherwise fit young women.

Massive pulmonary emboli are usually fatal before treatment is possible. Occasionally surgical intervention is possible. For the majority of patients treatment is by anticoagulation, initially with **heparin** followed by **warfarin**. This treatment is usually continued for some months and sometimes indefinitely where the risk factor persists.

ARTERIAL EMBOLI

These are usually small clots arising in the systemic circulation which occlude arteries of variable size depending on the size of the embolus. They may arise from abnormalities of the left atrium, heart valves, and endocardium, or from the walls of the larger arteries. They are seen in association with rheumatic valvular heart disease, subacute bacterial endocarditis, ischaemic heart disease, and atrial fibrillation.

The major organs affected are the brain, gastrointestinal tract, kidneys, and limbs. Emboli may cause transient symptoms with no permanent deficit or result in infarction of the tissue supplied by the occluded artery.

Treatment is aimed at preventing further emboli where applicable, removal of the embolus, and management of the complications. Anticoagulation may be indicated in certain circumstances.

Dental Significance

Oral anticoagulants, such as **warfarin** (*Marevan*$_{\text{GB}}$, *Coumadin*$_{\text{US}}$) prolong the clotting time by antagonism to vitamin K. Their action is potentiated by a number of hypnotics, analgesics, and antibiotics such as **barbiturates, salicylates, chloramphenicol** (*Chloromycetin*$_{GB,US}$ and *Kemicetine*$_{GB}$) and **metronidazole** (*Flagyl*$_{GB,US}$). These should be used with caution on patients being treated with anticoagulants. If extractions are contemplated, the patient's doctor should be consulted with regards to stopping treatment for a few days. Parenteral vitamin K in doses of 10 mg or more will reverse the action of anticoagulants in 24 hours.

EMPHYSEMA

There are two main types of emphysma.

(1) PAN-ACINAR

This is dilatation or destruction of the acini.

(2) CENTRILOBULAR

This is dilatation or destruction more proximal, involving the respiratory bronchioles.

Aetiology

Emphysema most commonly occurs with long-standing disease of the bronchi, bronchitis, asthma, or a combination of these conditions. It may relate to occupational exposure to dusts. Occasionally it develops as a primary disease.

The major symptom is dyspnoea, increasing with severity of the disease. Progression of symptoms is slow, taking years rather than months. Typically the patient with predominant emphysema is greatly distressed by shortness of breath whilst remaining pink ('pink puffer'). In contrast, the chronic bronchitic is less troubled by breathlessness though often deeply cyanosed ('blue bloater'). Usually the two conditions co-exist and symptoms of both are seen. In established disease the chest is over-inflated and chest expansion diminished.

Treatment consists of avoidance of harmful environmental factors such as smoke and dust, improvement of the airway by treating any bronchospasm, and prompt treatment of super-added infection. Respiratory exercises are valuable, enabling maximum use to be made of the remaining functional lung. The major complications are respiratory failure and heart failure from cor pulmonale.

Dental Significance

General anaesthetics are to be avoided.

ENCEPHALITIS

This is inflammation of the brain most commonly complicating viral infections, such as herpes, influenza, mumps, and measles. It is a serious complication characterized by fever, headache, vomiting, confusion, convulsions, coma, and occasionally death. Permanent brain damage of varying degree occurs in a significant number of patients and epilepsy may result.

In most cases there is no specific treatment though antiviral agents are sometimes used.

Treatment is supportive and symptomatic.

Dental Significance

None.

ENDOCARDITIS, see HEART DISEASE (Infective), SUBACUTE BACTERIAL ENDOCARDITIS.

ENTERIC FEVER, see TYPHOID

EPIDEMIC MYALGIA, see BORNHOLM'S DISEASE.

EPILEPSY

This is a recurrent disturbance of the electrical activity of the brain resulting in symptoms which include impairment of consciousness, convulsive movements, sensory abnormalities, and psychic disturbances. Epileptic attacks may be classified in the following way.

(1) GENERAL EPILEPSY

(a) Grand Mal

Typically there is an initial aura, followed by the tonic stage with loss of consciousness, cessation of respiration, and cyanosis. After this the clonic stage occurs with convulsive movements affecting the trunk, limbs, jaw, and tongue; in this stage the patient may froth at the mouth, bite the tongue, and be incontinent. Coma follows, lasting minutes to hours. Recovery is often accompanied by headache and occasionally post-epileptic automatism.

(b) Petit Mal

These attacks consist of brief periods of loss of consciousness when the patient stops what he is doing or saying for a few seconds then carries on.

(2) FOCAL EPILEPSY

This results from focal electrical discharges, the clinical manifestations depending on the site involved. They may be so minor as to pass unnoticed. Temporal lobe epilepsy results from electrical discharge in the temporal lobe resulting in organized movements, sensations, or emotions.

STATUS EPILEPTICUS

This is a serious complication of epilepsy where recurrent attacks occur in close succession without recovery of consciousness. Unless treated promptly this may lead to permanent brain damage or death.

Epilepsy may follow brain damage from any cause, trauma, cerebrovascular accidents, infection, or malignancy, but most commonly there is no obvious cause.

Management of grand mal. The aim is to prevent fits, by suppressing the abnormal electrical activity. The same range of drugs is used to treat both general and focal fits. **Phenytoin** (*Epanutin*$_{GB}$, *Dilantin*$_{US}$) and **carbamazepine** (*Tegretol*$_{GB,US}$) are drugs of choice, the latter being preferred in focal epilepsy. The use of the more sedative drugs such as **phenobarbitone** (*Luminal*$_{GB}$) and **primidone** (*Mysoline*$_{GB,US}$) is usually unnecessary. For petit mal **ethosuximide** (*Emeside*$_{GB}$ and *Zarontin*$_{GB,US}$) and **sodium valproate** (*Epilim*$_{GB}$, *Depakene*$_{US}$) are drugs of choice.

Status epilepticus should be treated with intravenous **diazepam** (*Valium*$_{GB,US}$) or **clonazepam** (*Rivotril*$_{GB}$). Care is required because of the risk of respiratory depression. **Diazepam** is given by slow intravenous injection initially up to 20 mg, watching the respiratory rate. This dose can be increased if there is no sign of respiratory depression. If this fails, intramuscular **paraldehyde** may be used (5–10 ml, not more than 5 ml in any one site) and arrangements made for urgent referral to hospital.

Dental Significance

There are no contra-indications to routine dentistry in epileptics. For those who suffer from grand mal loose-fitting partial dentures are inadvisable. Anaesthetic agents may be administered to epileptics in the dental surgery.

Fibrous hyperplasia of the gingivae occurs in 50 per cent of patients treated with **phenytoin** (*Epanutin*$_{GB}$, *Dilantin*$_{US}$). It seems to be unrelated to dosage but is commoner in the young. The underlying mechanism is not understood but meticulous plaque control helps to reduce the problem.

If a dentist is called to a patient having an attack of 'grand mal' epilepsy he should seek assistance to hold the patient on his side on the floor. If possible a dental prop or wedge of rubber or wood should be held between the patient's teeth, and he should be restrained from damaging himself until the clonic stage has passed. He should then be kept warm and allowed to rest until full consciousness has returned. Epileptics will know about their condition and are embarrassed by over-zealous and unnecessary after-care. Provided cyanosis was not prolonged and the patient is fully recovered and uninjured he or she may be allowed to return home.

EPILOIA, see TUBEROUS SCLEROSIS.

ERYSIPELAS

This is a skin infection caused by a group A streptococcus. It usually involves the face and head but may occur elsewhere beginning as an abrupt fever. A zone of redness and oedema occurs commonly on the bridge of the nose or around wounds, trauma sites, or an area of dermatitis. The facial lesion may spread to involve most of the face. Treatment is with **penicillin.**

Dental Significance

The condition is not of dental origin but dentists should recognize it as patients may consult them, thinking it is.

ERYTHEMA ANNULARE

This is a pink papule on the skin which enlarges to form a ring with a flattened centre up to 8 cm in diameter. It occurs on the buttocks, thighs, and upper arms. It is associated with malignancy.

Dental Significance

None.

ERYTHEMA MULTIFORME

This condition, mostly seen in young adults, is a reaction pattern in the skin and mucous membrane causing erythematous lesions which may be oedematous or bullous, darkening with age to give the characteristic target lesions. It has been associated with infections such as herpes simplex, with vaccination, drugs, and malignancy but in one-third of cases the cause is not known. The condition may present as a minor disease with few lesions or as a major life-threatening disease (see STEVENS–JOHNSON SYNDROME).

Dental Significance

The condition may present to the dentist as haemorrhagic bullae round the lips and in the mouth which quickly break down to ulcers. Among the drugs, used in dentistry, which are thought to be responsible factors are: **barbiturates, carbamazepine** (*Tegretol*$_{\text{GB,US}}$), **penicillin,** and **sulphonamides** (*Bactrim*$_{\text{GB,US}}$ and *Septrin*$_{\text{GB}}$). The condition is self-limiting but topical steroids in the form of **hydrocortisone** pellets (*Corlan*$_{\text{GB}}$) four times daily after meals, or **triamcinolone** (*Adcortyl*$_{\text{GB}}$, *Kenalog*$_{\text{US}}$) in orobase, will be helpful.

ERYTHEMA NODOSUM

This is considered to be a hypersensitivity vasculitis resulting in painful red nodules one or more centimetres in diameter. Most commonly these occur on the legs but are also seen on the arms. The condition is associated with infections such as tuberculosis, leprosy, and streptococcal infections; with sarcoid, inflammatory bowel disease, and with such drugs as **sulphonamides**. It is self-limiting. Treatment involves management of the underlying cause and treatment of symptoms.

Dental Significance

None.

F

FALLOT'S TETRALOGY, see HEART DISEASE (Congenital).

FAMILIAL PERIODIC PARALYSIS

This condition is characterized by recurrent attacks of flaccid weakness usually associated with hypokalaemia but occasionally hyperkalaemia. It is described in families with an autosomal dominant pattern of inheritance. Sporadic cases are seen. Diagnosis is based on a typical history and abnormal potassium levels in the serum.

Treatment of hypokalaemia is with oral potassium chloride, 5 to 10 g. Recovery is usual in ½ hour but may take hours. Hyperkalaemic paralysis requires an infusion of glucose and insulin. As a preventative treatment **acetazolamide** (*Diamox*$_{GB,US}$) has been found effective in both hyper- and hypokalaemic paralysis.

Dental Significance

None.

FARMER'S LUNG, see PNEUMOCONIOSIS.

FIBROCYSTIC DISEASE, see CYSTIC FIBROSIS.

FOOT AND MOUTH DISEASE

This virus disease is highly infectious among cattle, sheep, and pigs but seldom contracted by humans. The incubation period is 2–5 days and painful vesicles occur in the mouth and spread to other parts of the body, notably palms of hands and soles of feet. Diagnosis can be confirmed by laboratory examination of fluid from the vesicles.

Dental Significance

Though painful, the disease is not dangerous and clears up in 1–2 weeks. Secondary infection of oral lesions can be prevented by use of **erythromycin** mouthwash (5 ml of Erythroped$_{GB}$ or *Ilosone*$_{GB,US}$ 25 mg to 1 ml) in children and **tetracycline** and **amphotericin** mouthwash (5 ml *Mysteclin*$_{GB,US}$) in adults.

FRIEDREICH'S ATAXIA

This heredo-familial disorder presents in the first or second decade with unsteadiness, clumsiness, dysarthria, then weakness and ataxia. Additional features on examination include nystagmus, absent knee and ankle jerks, extensor plantar reflexes, optic atrophy, pes cavus, scoliosis, and cardiac arrhythmias.

There is no treatment.

Dental Significance

None.

G

GALL BLADDER DISEASE, see BILIARY DISEASE.

GALLSTONES, see BILIARY DISEASE.

GASTRIC ULCER, see PEPTIC ULCER.

GASTRITIS

G

ACUTE GASTRITIS

This is a diffuse inflammation of the gastric mucosa resulting from various factors: alcohol, aspirin, and anti-inflammatory drugs. In most cases the cause is poorly understood. The symptoms are epigastric discomfort, nausea, and loss of appetite.

Treatment is similar to that of peptic ulceration.

ATROPHIC GASTRITIS

This is a chronic inflammation of the stomach resulting in gastric mucosal atrophy and achlorhydria, leading to pernicious anaemia.

Dental Significance

With atrophy of the gastric mucosa, secretion of intrinsic factor (of Castle) is diminished and this results in failure to absorb vitamin B12. Together with a megaloblastic anaemia the patient may suffer from a painful atrophic glossitis and recurrent oral ulceration.

GASTROENTERITIS

This is a clinical syndrome of diarrhoea and vomiting associated with gastrointestinal infection, either viral or bacterial. Most attacks last no more than a few days and are self-limiting. They commonly result from ingestion of contaminated water or food where hygiene is poor. Symptomatic treatment is usually all that is required. In general antibiotics do not affect the course of the disease and may delay clearance of the organism from the gut. Some studies have suggested that prophylactic use of broad-spectrum antibiotics such as **sulphatriad** (a compound **sulphonamide**) may reduce attack rate. The best preventative measures are largely common sense: when in areas of poor hygiene, boil drinking water, avoid salad, peel fruit, don't buy it precut, and take great care with personal hygiene.

Dental Significance

None.

GAUCHER'S DISEASE

This is a familial disorder resulting in an abnormal accumulation of glyco-cerebrocides in the reticuloendothelial cells. Three syndromes are recognized.

(1) a chronic adult form with hypersplenism, bone lesions, pingueculae and skin pigmentation—this is the most common form;
(2) an acute neuropathic form seen in infancy, and usually fatal;
(3) a juvenile form combining features of the chronic form with progressive neurological dysfunctions.

There is no specific treatment.

Dental Significance

Radiotranslucent areas have been reported in the mandible. Nasal and gingival bleeding may occur, with excessive haemorrhage following dental extractions.

GERMAN MEASLES, see RUBELLA.

GIANT URTICARIA, see ANGIONEUROTIC OEDEMA.

GIARDIASIS

This is a gastrointestinal infection caused by the protozoan *Giardia lamblia.* It occurs worldwide, not just in the tropics but in any area of poor hygiene. Many holidaymakers in Leningrad seem to contract the infection. It may present as an acute illness with diarrhoea, nausea, abdominal pain, and vomiting or as a chronic diarrhoeal illness.

Diagnosis depends on demonstrating cysts in the stool or the protozoa in jejunal juice.

Treatment. The drug of choice is **metronidazole** (*Flagyl*$_{\text{GB,US}}$) 400 mg 8-hourly for 7 days.

Dental Significance

None.

GILBERT'S SYNDROME

The importance of this condition is in differentiating it from other causes of jaundice because it is entirely benign and of no clinical significance once correctly diagnosed. The important features are mild jaundice and a modest rise in unconjugated bilirubin in the blood. The condition is seen in between 3 and 7 per cent of the general population and is more common in men. It is due to a congenital defect in hepatic bile clearance from the circulation. The cause is not known.

Dental Significance

None.

GLANDULAR FEVER, see INFECTIOUS MONONUCLEOSIS.

GLAUCOMA

Glaucoma is a rise in intra-ocular pressure sufficient to cause degeneration of the optic disc and visual field defects. It is a leading cause of acquired blindness estimated to occur in 2 per cent of adults over 40.

The condition may be primary (open angle), secondary, or congenital. Primary glaucoma is a slowly progressive bilateral disease of insidious onset. Treatment is usually medical and prognosis good. Untreated, complete blindness results. Congenital glaucoma is due to anterior segment anomalies. Symptoms are dramatic with the onset of sudden severe pain, nausea, and vomiting with blurring of vision. Attacks may be precipitated by mydriatics such as atropine. Such drugs should not be used if glaucoma is suspected.

Treatment is with oral **glycerine** and **pilocarpine.** Iridectomy is indicated when medical treatment fails.

Dental Significance

A dentist should always enquire if a patient suffers from glaucoma before giving **atropine** in any form.

GLOMERULONEPHRITIS, see RENAL DISEASE.

GONORRHOEA

This is a venereal disease due to the gonococcus *Neisseria gonorrhoeae*. It is usually acquired by coitus with an infected person. The incubation period of 3–10 days is followed by dysuria, a purulent urethral discharge, and tender groin glands. In men the prostate and seminal vesicles may be involved and in women Bartholin's gland, the uterus, and fallopian tubes may become infected leading to permanent sterility. Septic arthritis may complicate the infection. Infection does not convey immunity.

Treatment is with **procaine penicillin** with **probenecid** (*Benemid*$_{GB,US}$). However, resistant strains of the gonococcus are now common, accounting for the increased failure rate of conventional treatment.

Dental Significance

Gonorrhoeal stomatitis or tonsillitis can result from direct infection through oral sex with an infected partner, by auto-transfer from a patient's genital infection, or as part of a disseminated gonococcal infection. Painful inflammation and oedema of the mucous membrane is usual: ulceration less common. Arthritis of the temporomandibular joint is a rare complication.

Diagnosis is not possible from a direct smear and culture from a swab of exudate is necessary.

Treatment is with IM **procaine penicillin** 600 mg daily and **probenecid** (*Benemid*$_{GB,US}$) 250 mg twice daily for 1 week.

GOUT

This clinical syndrome results from a rise in the serum uric acid level. The cause of the rise may be an excessive synthesis as is postulated in primary or genetic gout, and as is seen in conditions of excessive tissue turnover, lymphomas, and leukaemia. The alternative cause is reduced renal clearance most commonly seen in renal failure, and as a complication of the use of certain drugs, e.g. thiazide diuretics.

The main clinical feature is acute arthritis most commonly effecting the first metatarsophalangeal joints. Crystal deposits are seen in the skin or gouty tophi. The condition is complicated by renal crystal deposits leading to infection and renal damage.

Treatment of the acute attacks is with **indomethacin** (*Indocid*$_{GB}$, *Indocin*$_{US}$). Preventative treatment involves avoidance of drugs known to precipitate gout and the use of the xanthine oxidase inhibitor **allopurinol** (*Zyloric*$_{GB}$, *Lopurin*$_{US}$, *Zyloprim*$_{US}$).

Dental Significance

The arthritis of gout may involve the temporomandibular joint, and if so a soft bite block will make the patient more comfortable.

GRAVE'S DISEASE, see THYROID DISEASE.

GUILLAIN-BARRÉ SYNDROME

This syndrome is an acute neuropathy, predominantly motor, of uncertain aetiology. Most probably there is a cell-mediated immune response provoked by certain viral infections, and directed at normal peripheral myelin. There is frequently a history of an infective illness, viral in nature, in the preceding few weeks. Progressive weakness occurs over 2–3 weeks commonly affecting the lower limbs first, but the arms and cranial nerves are frequently affected and involvement of muscles of respiration may necessitate ventilation.

Recovery is usual, but 20 per cent of patients are left with residual disability. The cerebrospinal fluid protein is usually raised though the cell count is normal.

There is no specific treatment. Management consists of careful nursing, physiotherapy, and a continuous awareness of the possible need of artificial ventilation.

Dental Significance

Weakness in muscles of mastication, with difficulty in chewing, has been reported.

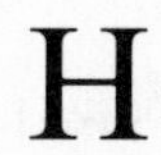

HAEMOCHROMATOSIS, see LIVER DISEASE.

HAEMOPHILIA, CHRISTMAS DISEASE and VON WILLEBRAND'S DISEASE

These inherited blood dyscrasias are caused by a missing factor in the complicated process of blood-clotting whose absence results in persistent haemorrhage. Factor VIII is missing in haemophilia, Factor IX in Christmas disease, and Factor VIII together with VW Factor in Von Willebrand's disease.

Dental Significance

At the present day in the United Kingdom it is to be expected that all sufferers will be under the care and guidance of a haemophilia centre and dental treatment should only be undertaken after consulting them.

Providing the patient has not built up a titre of antibodies against the replacement factor, most procedures of conservative dentistry can be carried out after the patient has received an administration (intravenously) of the missing factor approximately 1 hour before treatment, supplemented by an anti-fibrinolytic and where necessary an antibiotic.

Nerve block anaesthesia must be avoided but infiltration injections of local anaesthetic are permissible, and this can be supplemented, when required, by intravenous sedation or relative analgesia. Dangerous haematomas in the floor of the mouth can result from use of saliva ejectors and bitewing X-ray holders, and the floor of the mouth should be protected with gauze when using these.

Cavity preparation should be undertaken with extra care to avoid laceration of the gingiva and in root treatment the dentist must avoid reaming through the apex.

Extractions and oral surgery of anything but the most minor sort must be carried out in hospital in full consultation with the haemophilia centre. Tissue trauma should be kept to a minimum and plugs, packs, and tight suturing avoided.

The prescription of postoperative analgesics containing **aspirin** is contra-indicated.

Because of frequent screening the risk of haemophiliacs being hepatitis carriers is less than it was, and they need not be automatically classed as high-risk patients in this respect. Treatment procedure should be based on their serological analysis (see Liver Disease—Hepatitis).

HAND, FOOT, AND MOUTH DISEASE

The disease is caused by infection with the Cocksackie A virus, has an incubation period of 3–6 days, and is seen mainly in young children. Painful ulcers occur in the mouth and vesicles on the palmar surface of the hands and plantar surface of the feet. There is usually mild pyrexia and malaise. The condition resolves in about 10 days. There is no treatment.

Dental Significance

Antiseptic lozenges containing a local anaesthetic will ease the patient's discomfort and prevent secondary infection. It is likely that the virus is present in exudate from the ulcers so care should be taken in sterilizing instruments and the rinse-out glass.

HANSEN'S DISEASE see LEPROSY

HASHIMOTO'S DISEASE, see THYROID DISEASE.

HEART DISEASE (Congenital)

ATRIAL SEPTAL DEFECT (ASD)

An ASD of the ostium secundum type is a common developmental cardiac abnormality resulting in a left-to-right heart shunt. It often gives rise to no symptoms until adult life when dyspnoea and palpitations due to extrasystoles or atrial fibrillation occur. The important complication is pulmonary hypertension which may lead to shunt reversal and cyanosis. The ostium premium ASD is much rarer and associated with mitral incompetence and left axis deviation on the ECG.

Treatment is surgical for moderate to large shunts and contra-indicated with severe pulmonary hypertension.

Dental Significance

Patients with open or repaired atrial defects should receive antibiotic cover for all procedures likely to cause a bacteraemia (see HEART DISEASE (infective), SUBACUTE BACTERIAL ENDOCARDITIS). With those having small or repaired defects it is safe to give a general anaesthetic in the surgery, but reduced exercise tolerance requires the administration of anaesthetics in hospital.

FALLOT'S TETRALOGY

The anatomical features of this condition are pulmonary stenosis, a high ventricular septal defect, an overriding aorta, and right ventricular hypertrophy. It is the commonest form of congenital cyanotic heart disease. Complete surgical repair is the treatment of choice.

Dental Significance

Antibiotic cover is mandatory for all dental procedures likely to cause a bacteraemia (see HEART DISEASE (Infective), SUBACUTE BACTERIAL ENDOCARDITIS). General anaesthetics should only be administered in hospital.

PATENT DUCTUS ARTERIOSUS

This is a developmental abnormality where a foetal channel between the aorta and main pulmonary artery persists. It is commonly asymptomatic but if large may lead to dyspnoea and palpitations. Examination reveals a loud continuous murmur (Gibson, or machinery murmur). Pulmonary hypertension and bacterial endocarditis are complications of the untreated condition. Treatment is surgical and curative if performed before complications occur.

Dental Significance

Antibiotic cover for procedures likely to cause a bacteraemia is probably wise, but for patients with this defect untreated or treated the risk is small (see HEART DISEASE (Infective), SUBACUTE BACTERIAL ENDOCARDITIS). A small asymptomatic patent ductus, or one which has been successfully closed, does not mitigate against general anaesthetics in the surgery.

VENTRICULAR SEPTAL DEFECT

This defect may involve the membranous or muscular part of the septum. Small defects produce no disability and are compatible with a normal life, while larger ones lead to heart failure, the degree of shunt depending on the size of the defect. Auscultation reveals a loud pansystolic murmur. The major complications are pulmonary hypertension and bacterial endocarditis. Pyogenic infections and dental procedures should be covered by antibiotics. Patients with small shunts can lead normal lives while surgery is the treatment of choice for larger defects.

Dental Significance

All dental procedures likely to cause a bacteraemia should receive antibiotic cover (see HEART DISEASE (Infective), SUBACUTE BACTERIAL ENDOCARDITIS). General anaesthetics should be administered in hospital.

HEART DISEASE (Dysrythmias)

ATRIAL FIBRILLATION

This results from multiple ectopic foci discharging rapidly, producing very rapid atrial rates, 400/minute or more. The ventricles are unable to respond to this rate and respond at a variable rate between 60 and 200 due to variable electrical block.

Most commonly it results from ischaemic heart disease but may be due to thyrotoxicosis, pneumonia, or valvular heart disease.

Ventricular rate is controlled with **digoxin**. Systemic embolization is the main hazard. Heart failure may complicate uncontrolled fibrillation.

Dental Significance

Aspirating syringes and local anaesthetics without adrenaline should be used in these patients. Antibiotic cover will not be required unless there is a history of rheumatic or congenital heart disease, in which case it should be given for 'at-risk' procedures as described in HEART DISEASE (Infective), SUBACUTE BACTERIAL ENDOCARDITIS. Unless the condition is fully controlled, anaesthetics should only be administered in hospital.

PAROXYSMAL ATRIAL TACHYCARDIA

Commonly atrial or supraventricular, these paroxysms, arising from a single ectopic focus, come on suddenly and usually result in a pulse rate between 150 and 220 per minute. The duration is from minutes to days. Although sometimes associated with underlying heart disease, commonly the heart is normal. They occur at any age and may be associated with anomolous atrio-ventricular conduction as in the Wolf–Parkinson–White (WPW) syndrome, where premature ventricular excitation occurs due to conduction via an anomalous pathway to the ventricles. The ECG may be normal or show the characteristic short P–R interval. In the absence of underlying heart disease the prognosis is excellent. Treatment consists of reassurance. Usually attacks cease spontaneously but carotid sinus massage is sometimes effective in arresting the attack. When prolonged antidysrhythmic agents such as **verapamil** (*Cordilox*$_{\text{GB}}$) are indicated.

Dental Significance

There are no contra-indications to routine dental treatment. General anaesthetics may be administered to patients who suffer from this condition provided there is no underlying heart disease and the pulse is normal at the time. Commensurate treatment with **verapamil** may potentiate the hypotensive effect of anaesthetic agents.

HEART BLOCK

The term 'heart block' describes a situation where the conduction of electrical excitation from the atria is delayed at the junctional tissues (the AV node and His bundle). On the ECG the P–R interval is the time taken for the impulse to travel from the atria across the junctional tissue and down the ventricular bundles. In its mildest form (first-degree heart block) the P–R interval is abnormally prolonged (greater than 0.2 seconds). As conduction deteriorates, periodic impulses fail to cross to the ventricles and no ventricular beat occurs (second-degree block). In its most extreme form (third-degree block, complete heart block, or AV dissociation) no impulses pass from atria to ventricles and both beat independently of one another.

The commonest cause of heart block is ischaemic heart disease though it may result from viral infection, infiltrative disease such as amyloid, collagen disorders, cardiomyopathies, and occasionally it may be congenital. The prognosis of first-and second-degree heart block is favourable though this clearly depends on the underlying cause. The outcome in complete heart block is unpredictable and because of the high risk of cardiac standstill or ventricular fibrillation leading to Stokes–Adams attacks, any of which may be fatal, cardiac pacing is usually recommended. In the presence of Stokes–Adams attacks pacing is a matter of urgency, a temporary pacemaker being inserted until a permanent pacemaker can be implanted.

Cardiac pacemakers

Transvenous endocardial pacing is the method used for temporary pacing and the transvenous route is favoured for permanent pacing also. The two principal modes of pacing are fixed rate, when pacing is preset and occurs independently of intrinsic heart rate, and demand pacing when the pacemaker fires only when the ventricular rate falls below a predetermined level. The latter method is safer and the preferred method.

Dental Significance

Research has shown that diathermy and the magnetostrictive types of ultrasonic scalers can affect the function of pacemakers if in close proximity, and their use is therefore inadvisable. Though the risk is not high, antibiotic cover should be given to patients with pacemakers for procedures likely to cause a bacteraemia (see HEART DISEASE (Infective), SUBACUTE BACTERIAL ENDOCARDITIS).

General anaesthetics should be conducted in hospital.

STOKES–ADAMS ATTACK

This is a sudden loss of consciousness due to transient circulatory arrest resulting from ventricular asystole or tachycardia. It is almost invariably associated with underlying ischaemic heart disease particularly when complete heart block is present. Attacks may be infrequent or multiple in rapid succession. When associated with complete heart block permanent cardiac pacing is indicated.

Dental Significance

General anaesthetics are to be avoided, and if essential administered in hospital.

HEART DISEASE (Infective)

SUBACUTE BACTERIAL ENDOCARDITIS

This is the commonest form of endocarditis, and *Streptococcus viridans* the commonest organism. Infection may occur in any patient with a cardiac abnormality who has a bacteraemia. Although relatively rare it is an important condition because it carries a high mortality rate. This results in part from the non-specific early symptoms which are often overlooked, leading to delay in diagnosis. Specific symptoms are a result of emboli from valve cusp vegetations lodging in cerebral and peripheral vessels, and from valvular destruction leading to heart failure. Important clinical features are: fever, anaemia, splinter haemorrhage, haematuria, splenomegaly, and changing heart murmurs. A high ESR and a normochromic anaemia support the diagnosis, which is confirmed by blood cultures.

Antibiotic therapy depends on the organism and its sensitivity. Bactericidal antibiotics must be used, **penicillin** being the drug of choice for *Strep. viridans*. Treatment is classically intravenous and for 6 weeks though in some circumstances, where the organism is identified and sensitive to antibiotics, oral therapy may be justified.

Dental Significance

Extractions and some other dental procedures would appear to be important predisposing factors in this condition. Having said that, endocarditis following dental treatment is rare, only occurring in a small proportion of 'at-risk' patients after dental treatment. However, in view of the mortality of the disease, it is the duty of dentists to take reasonable measures towards its prevention.

It is important to identify high-risk patients. They fall into six groups:

(1) patients with any congenital heart disease;
(2) patients with rheumatic fever or post-rheumatic valvular heart disease;
(3) patients with prosthetic heart valves;
(4) patients with biscuspid aortic valves;
(5) debilitated and immunosuppressed patients;
(6) patients with cardiac pacemakers.

The dental procedures considered liable to cause endocarditis, and which warrant prophylactic antibiotic cover are: tooth extraction, deep scaling and periodontal surgery, and root-filling procedures where there is danger of forcing infected debris through the apex. The recommended prophylaxis is **amoxycillin** 3 g orally, 1 hour beforehand. For patients allergic to **penicillin**, oral **erythromycin** should be given in two doses of 2 g each, taken 3 hours before and 1 hour after dental treatment. Where general anaesthesia is needed intramuscular **amoxycillin** or **ampicillin** should be given 1 g an hour beforehand or **erythromycin** (where indicated) at the time of induction.

Patients with prosthetic valves may require additional cover with a second antibiotic such as **gentamycin**, and should be referred to hospital for 'at-risk' dental procedures.

Half the adult dose is given to children under 10 years and a quarter the dose under 5 years.

(The recommendations of the American Heart Association (1977) are that 1,000,000 units of **crystalline penicillin** and 600,000 units of **procaine penicillin** be given intramuscularly or

2 g of **penicillin V** by mouth 1 hour before operation, and then 500 mg **penicillin V** by mouth 6-hourly for 2 days. For patients with prosthetic heart valves the initial dose must be intramuscular and include 1 g of **streptomycin. Vancomycin** is the alternative antibiotic for those allergic to **penicillin**, and dosage for children appropriately scaled down).

HEART DISEASE (Ischaemic)

ANGINA PECTORIS

This term describes the symptom of myocardial ischaemia. It results when the heart muscle becomes critically short of oxygen, usually due to coronary artery atheroma. It may be aggravated by anaemia and anoxia. It is usually brought on by exercise but may occur unrelated to activity (unstable angina).

The main lines of treatment are:

(1) vasodilator drugs such as short and long acting nitrates, e.g. **glyceryl trinitrate** and **isosorbide dinitrate**
(2) beta-adrenoceptor blocking drugs which reduce cardiac work, e.g. **propranolol**.

MYOCARDIAL INFARCTION

More than ¼ million heart attacks occur each year in Britain and 40 per cent of patients die during the 4 weeks following their heart attack. Twenty-five per cent of these deaths are instantaneous. The cause of death is usually ventricular fibrillation. The pain from myocardial infarction is similar to anginal pain but very much more severe and persistent; however, very occasionally myocardial infarction is painless.

Dental Significance

Patients with a history of angina pectoris or myocardial infarction may be treated in a general dental practice with a few precautions. (When a patient has suffered a myocardial infarction surgical procedures should be delayed for 3 months if possible.)

General anaesthetics should be avoided, and painful conservative work and surgery carried out with local anaesthesia. A local anaesthetic solution without a vasoconstrictor should be employed, and intravenous injection avoided by use of an aspirating syringe. Care to avoid anxiety and stress is important, and oral or intravenous sedatives should be used where necessary.

Patients who use **nitrites** or **nitrates** to ease their symptoms should bring the drugs into the surgery with them.

If on anticoagulant therapy (**warfarin** or other anticoagulants) extractions or other surgery must only be undertaken after consultation with the patient's doctor or specialist. If the patient's life is not put at risk thereby, the anticoagulant treatment must be discontinued or reduced prior to surgery and a clotting time or prothrombin estimation checked to make sure that these figures are within normal limits.

CARDIAC ARREST

This is most commonly due to myocardial infarction but may occasionally complicate hypoxia due to an anaesthetic accident. Asystole may occur but more commonly the arrest results from ventricular fibrillation. Though the diagnosis is usually obvious, cardiac arrest is recognized by the following features: collapse, loss of consciousness, pallor, loss of pulses, and apnoea.

Management

Speed is essential; irreversible brain damage results within 3–5 minutes of arrest. The following manoeuvres should be carried out:

(1) lay the patient flat on the floor, face upwards;
(2) clear airway, remove dentures, loosen collar, insert airway if available, send assistant to call for ambulance;
(3) apply sharp blow with the hand to the lower sternum—in the case of a dysrhythmia this may restart the heart;
(4) commence external cardiac massage and mouth to mouth respiration. Place flat of right hand over lower half of sternum, place left hand on top of right hand, kneel beside patient, deliver five forcible thrusts to the chest at approximately 1-second intervals. Ventilate by closing the patient's nostrils with finger and thumb, inhaling deeply, and exhaling through patient's mouth.

This sequence of events should be repeated until assistance comes. Ventilation is more effective using an airway and ambu bag and preferably oxygen.

HENOCH–SCHONLEIN PURPURA (Anaphylactoid)

This is a syndrome consisting of purpura, painful joint swelling, abdominal pain, blood in the stools, and haematuria. The pathology shows widespread inflammation of small blood vessels with the histological appearance of a hypersensitivity reaction, the precise cause of which is not clear. It occurs mainly in children, frequently following an upper respiratory tract infection. There is no specific treatment. The course is usually benign, lasting 6–8 weeks, but a relapsing course may be seen and 5–10 per cent of patients may develop chronic nephritis.

Dental Significance

None.

HEPATITIS, see LIVER DISEASE.

HEPATO-LENTICULAR DEGENERATION, see LIVER DISEASE.

HEREDITARY HAEMORRHAGIC TELANGIECTASIA (Oslar/Rendu/Weber syndrome)

This is a condition characterized by telangiectases on the face, lips, tongue, fingers, alimentary tract, and nasal mucosa. Inheritance is as an autosomal dominant. The lesions increase in number with age and bleeding becomes an increasing problem in adult life with troublesome nosebleeds and gastro-intestinal haemorrhage resulting in iron deficiency anaemia. There is no specific treatment besides haemostasis and replacement therapy, though oestrogens may be of value in troublesome epistaxis.

Dental Significance

If the telangiectases are present on the lips or in the mouth, care must be taken to avoid damaging them, as haemorrhage may be profuse.

HERPES SIMPLEX

PRIMARY HERPES

This is an acute infection, usually seen in childhood or adolescence, caused by the herpes virus. The condition is characterized by pyrexia; enlargement of lymph nodes; and a crop of vesicles on the gingiva, buccal mucosa, and lips. These rapidly break down to small ulcers and are extremely painful. Vesicles may occur in other parts of the body. Frequently the condition is seen in patients with immunity disorders or those being treated with immunosuppressants.

In children treatment is with **erythromycin** suspension (*Erythroped*$_{GB}$, *Ilosone*$_{GB,US}$), used as a mouthwash four times daily (5 ml containing 125 mg). This should be held in the mouth as long as possible before being swallowed or spat out. For adults a **tetracycline** and **amphotericin** mouthwash (*Mysteclin*$_{GB,US}$), 5 ml four times daily, is advised. Though ineffective against the causative virus this prevents secondary infection. **Idoxuridine** 0.1 per cent in purified water can be applied to lesions on the lips and in the mouth, but has an unpleasant taste, and there is doubt whether it is of value in this form and at this stage of the condition. Recovery occurs over about a week.

RECURRENT HERPES

Recurrent attacks at the same site may occur over a period of years. There is no specific treatment though **idoxuridine** paint 5 per cent (*Herpid*$_{GB}$) may be applied to lesions on the skin and a 0.1 per cent solution of **idoxuridine** used as a mouthwash. **Erythromycin** reduces symptoms, possibly by treating any secondary infection.

Applications of **ether** to recurrent herpes labialis is claimed to hasten resolution, and **carbenoxolone** 2 per cent cream is said to be beneficial.

Dental Significance

Children with primary herpes may be brought to the dentist because of the gingivitis, which must be recognized and differentiated from acute ulcerative gingivitis.

By adult life most people have acquired an immunity to the virus and there is no real risk of infection from contact with herpetic patients. It is frequently mentioned that herpetic whitlows are an occupational hazard of dentists, but in their personal experience the authors have little evidence to support this.

HERPES ZOSTER (Shingles)

This condition, caused by the same virus as chicken pox, is due to infection of the posterior root ganglion resulting in severe pain and a vesicular skin eruption in the dermatome supplied by the corresponding posterior root. Occasionally in people with malignant disease or impaired immunity, infection can become generalized and resemble chicken pox. The complications of herpes zoster are more severe in older people. Involvement of the ophthalmic nerve results in corneal lesions which may cause impairment of vision. Geniculate ganglion involvement results in vesicular formation in the pinna over the mastoid and sometimes in the fauces. It can cause facial palsy and loss of taste over the anterior two-thirds of the tongue. Paralysis elsewhere occurs, and though uncommon, encephalitis and myelitis are both described.

Early treatment with steroids may shorten the attack and prevent the post-herpetic pain. However, post-herpetic neuralgia often remains the major problem and is extremely difficult to treat. **Carbamazepine** (*Tegretol*$_{GB,US}$) is the most effective drug with which to treat the condition, but sometimes neurosurgical intervention is required.

Dental Significance

When the second and third divisions of the trigeminal nerve are involved the lesions appear on the face and sometimes on the lips and in the mouth. On the face and lips **idoxuridine** paint 5 per cent (*Herpid*$_{GB}$) should be applied to the lesions four times a day in the prevesicular stage. On the moist surface of the lips and inner cheek **triamcinolone** acetonide (*Adcortyl*$_{GB}$, *Kenalog*$_{US}$) in orobase, will help; while a four times daily mouthwash of **tetracyclin** and **amphotericin** (*Mysteclin*$_{GB,US}$) will help to prevent secondary infection.

Usually adults have acquired immunity to the virus in childhood. Thus, although it is possible to develop chicken pox from contact with herpes zoster, in practice this is extremely uncommon. Herpes zoster results from reactivation of previously acquired virus. It does not result from contact either with chicken pox or others with herpes zoster. Thus, although a child could contract chicken pox from a dentist suffering with herpes zoster, a dentist would not contract herpes zoster from a patient with either chicken pox or herpes.

HIATUS HERNIA

This is herniation of part of the stomach upwards through the diaphragmatic hiatus into the chest. Herniation may be either sliding or rolling. The former is most common and is the major cause of symptoms: acid reflux and heartburn. Ulceration and stricture formation of the oesophagus complicate long-standing acid reflux. The principles of treatment are avoidance of the horizontal position, reduction in acid secretion, avoidance of smoking and obesity. Surgery may be indicated where medical treatment fails.

Dental Significance

Acid reflux into the oesophagus may result in referred pain being experienced in the throat and molar teeth. Cases have been reported where repeated regurgitation of gastric acid into the mouth has caused enamel erosion of posterior teeth.

Patients suffering from this condition dislike being treated in the supine position, and the dentist should appreciate their problem and adapt his methods to save them discomfort.

General anaesthetics should be administered in hospital.

HODGKIN'S DISEASE, see LYMPHOPROLIFERATIVE DISEASE.

HUNTINGTON'S CHOREA, see CHOREA.

HYPERALDOSTERONISM, see ADRENAL DISEASE.

HYPERGLYCAEMIA, see DIABETES MELLITUS.

HYPERLIPIDAEMIAS

Frederickson's classification divides these conditions into five types. Types I, III, and V are rare. Type IV is the commonest, accounting for 35–50 per cent of all hyperlipidaemias. The serum is turbid, triglycerides raised, but cholesterol normal. It is associated with obesity and diabetes and the clinical features include xanthomata, lipaemia retinalis, and atherosclerosis. Treatment consists of a low-carbohydrate diet. Types IIa and IIb constitute 40 per cent of the cases seen. Here the serum is clear but cholesterol is raised. Xanthomata are present in IIa but not IIb. Both are associated with atherosclerosis and type IIb with diabetes mellitus.

Treatment of both involves a low cholesterol and low saturated fat diet.

Dental Significance

The association of the condition with diabetes mellitus and ischaemic heart disease should be borne in mind by the dentist. Local anaesthetics without **adrenaline** should be used, and a medical opinion sought before administering a general anaesthetic.

Xanthelasmata on the upper eyelid are often of no significance, but occasionally may be associated with hyperlipidaemia.

HYPERTENSION

Most commonly this is primary or essential where no cause is known, but occasionally hypertension may be secondary to the following diseases: renal disease, Cushing's disease, Conn's syndrome, phaeochromocytoma, renal artery stenosis, and coarctation of the aorta.

Hypertension may cause few or no symptoms even when quite severe, and may only be discovered when the consequencs of long-standing hypertension develop, for example cerebrovascular and ischaemic heart disease and renal damage. Occasionally hypertension progresses rapidly to grossly elevated levels, giving rise to severe headache, vomiting, dizziness, breathlessness, and coma. In this type of hypertension, malignant hypertension, unless urgent treatment is instigated the mortality rate is high. In other forms of hypertension, recognition of its existence is important so that early treatment can be commenced to prevent complications. There is debate as to the level at which treatment is indicated but levels above 140/90 are generally felt to warrant treatment and studies have shown that treatment of mild hypertension reduces the incidence of cerebrovascular disease and probably cardiovascular disease as well, though the evidence for the latter is less clear at present. Blood pressure results from the interaction between cardiac output and peripheral vascular resistance, and treatment is aimed at reducing one or other of these.

Vasodilator drugs include **hydralazine** (*Apresoline*$_{GB,US}$) and **prazosin** (*Hypovase*$_{GB}$, *Minipress*$_{US}$). Centrally acting drugs include **methyldopa** (*Aldomet*$_{GB,US}$) and **clonidine** (*Catapres*$_{GB,US}$). Adrenergic neurone-blocking drugs include **guanethidine** (*Ismelin*$_{GB,US}$) and **bethanidine** (*Esbatal*$_{GB}$). Alpha-adrenergic blocking drugs include **phenoxybenzamine** (*Dibenyline*$_{GB}$, *Dibenzyline*$_{US}$), and **phentolamine** (*Rogitine*$_{GB}$, *Regitine*$_{US}$).

The most commonly used hypotensive agents are the beta-adrenoceptor blocking drugs of which there are now many on the market. In general these are freer of side-effects than many of the other hypotensive agents; no one agent seems clearly superior to another. Examples are **atenolol** (Tenormin$_{GB}$) and **metoprolol** (*Betaloc*$_{GB}$, *Lopresor*$_{GB,US}$).

Dental Significance

There are no contra-indications to routine dentistry for patients with hypertension or those taking antihypertensive drugs, provided local anaesthetics with adrenaline are avoided.

Unless the patient is being treated with **warfarin**, blood clotting will be normal, but some increased haemorrhage following dental extractions may be experienced.

General anaesthetics in the surgery may be administered to patients with mild hypertension or those in whom the blood pressure is controlled to 180/110 or less, but the blood pressure should be checked immediately prior to administration, immediately afterwards and before the patient leaves. Anaesthetic agents, which lower the blood pressure, may potentiate the action of antihypertensive drugs, and the patient should remain lying down until the blood pressure has returned to normal, or to its previous level.

I

IMPETIGO

Impetigo is a skin infection caused by streptococcal or mixed streptococcal and staphylococcal infection. The ostia of the pilosebaceous follicles or sweat ducts are involved, or breaks in the skin due to scratches or bites. It may be associated with scabies or pediculosis. The infection may originate from coccal infections involving the nose, ears, or eyes. The typical lesions consist of red raised spots topped with a yellowish-brown crust, most commonly on the face but also on the limbs and in the scalp. The condition frequently occurs in outbreaks affecting several members of the family or school.

Prompt treatment is required as the condition spreads rapidly. Children should be kept away from other children and use a separate towel. **Gentamycin** (*Genticin*$_{\mathrm{GB}}$, *Garamycin*$_{\mathrm{US}}$) cream applied three or four times daily is effective, but if widespread **flucloxacillin** (*Floxapen*$_{\mathrm{GB}}$) 125–250 mg four times daily should be given.

Dental Significance

If encountering the condition in a patient, dentists should take care not to pass on the infection via their hands or white coats.

INFARCTION, see HEART DISEASE (Ischaemic).

INFECTIOUS MONONUCLEOSIS (Glandular Fever)

This is an acute infectious disease caused by the Epstein-Barr virus (EBV). It is common in children and adolescents but occurs in older age groups. It spreads most rapidly under conditions of crowding and close physical contact. Distribution is worldwide. The incubation period is 30–50 days in adults but shorter, 4–14 days in young children.

Mild malaise, fatigue, and headache may occur during the 4–5 day prodromal phase. Initial clinical symptoms include fever, sore throat, and cervical lymphadenopathy. The sore throat may be severe with oedema of the pharynx and exudative tonsillitis lasting several days. Oedema may rarely become severe enough to threaten the airway. In addition to signs in the throat and gland enlargement splenomegaly commonly occurs and although hepatomegaly occurs less frequently, liver function tests are frequently abnormal and jaundice is seen in 5 per cent of patients.

Complications include aseptic meningitis, encephalitis, Bell's palsy, thrombocytopenic purpura, haemolytic anaemia, myocarditis, and pericarditis.

Diagnosis is confirmed by seeing atypical mononuclear cells in the peripheral blood picture and a positive Paul–Bunnell test.

Treatment is symptomatic. **Prednisolone** may be indicated where pharyngeal oedema is severe, and occasionally tracheostomy is necessary.

Dental Significance

Glandular fever should be suspected in children and adolescents who present with an intensely sore throat which is inflamed, oedematous, with small sloughs on the tonsils, and accompanied by fever and cervical adenitis. Less commonly there are ulcers in the mouth. Antibiotics are ineffective and a sensitivity rash may result from the administration of **ampicillin**.

At this stage the patient is infective and precautions such as face mask for dentist and assistant, and thorough sterilization of instruments and rinse-out glass, should be taken.

INFLUENZA

Influenza is an acute febrile illness of short duration with malaise, fever, generalized aches and pains, headache, often associated with the symptoms of an upper respiratory tract infection. The disease is most commonly caused by influenza viruses A or B. Influenza virus C causes sporadic mild illness. The incubation period is 2–3 days. The duration of the illness is usually 3–4 days. Influenza may be complicated by encephalomyelitis or secondary bacterial pneumonia.

Treatment. Prophylactic influenza vaccines have a proven protective value, lasting up to 1 year. Treatment of the disease is symptomatic. In general the prognosis is good but the infection can cause a high mortality rate amongst the elderly and those with chronic lung disease.

Dental Significance

By reason of their close face-to-face contact with patients, dentists are at risk of picking up 'flu which is spread by droplet infection. There is some doubt about the value of 'flu vaccine as a protection against the endemic disease, but when, as a result of an 'antigen shift', a pandemic breaks out a dentist is well advised to seek vaccine protection. He can, if he wishes, easily administer it to himself and will find clear instructions on the vial. It should not be given to anyone allergic to eggs.

INTRACRANIAL HAEMORRHAGE

Intracranial haemorrhage may result from rupture of veins, as is seen in subdural haematomas, or more commonly arteries, as in subarachnoid haemorrhage. Intracranial haemorrhage may also result from rupture of microaneurysms or cerebral angiomas and extradural haemorrhage from rupture of a meningeal artery.

EXTRADURAL HAEMATOMAS

These result from cranial trauma usually associated with fracture of the temporal bone and consequent rupture of the middle meningeal artery. Typically the patient recovers from the initial trauma only to lapse into unconsciousness with the development of the haematoma. This is a neurosurgical emergency of the first degree, death ensuing unless the bleeding is stopped and the clot evacuated promptly.

Dental Significance

Dentists seeing patients with traumatic injuries to the face and jaws must be alert to the possibility of a fracture of the skull occurring at the same time. Any patient who has been knocked unconscious, or who has retrograde amnesia and cannot remember the events leading up to the accident, should be referred to hospital for assessment.

SUBDURAL HAEMATOMAS

Although occasionally acute, following trauma, most commonly these are chronic resulting from rupture of cortical veins. Although trauma is suspected as a major cause, often there is no history of trauma or the trauma was only mild. Those particularly prone to subdurals are the elderly and those exposed to repeated head trauma such as alcoholics. Diagnosis may be difficult and is often missed. It depends on an awareness of the possibility in the face of vague and varied neurological features, personality change, fits, headaches, and variable level of consciousness. Confirmation comes from a CAT scan or angiography. Treatment is surgical but due to the chronic nature of the haematoma neurological recovery is often disappointing.

SUBARACHNOID HAEMORRHAGE

This is arterial bleeding into the subarachnoid space, usually due to spontaneous rupture of a cerebral aneurysm on the circle of Willis (Berry aneurysm). Symptoms are often dramatic with sudden onset of severe headache sometimes associated with loss of consciousness and followed by meningism and photophobia. One-third of patients die in the first attack, but the prognosis is greatly improved in those who survive the initial 2 weeks.

Treatment is surgical if the aneurysm is accessible.

INTRACEREBRAL HAEMORRHAGE

When intracranial bleeding occurs within the brain substance, destruction of brain tissue and consequent neurological deficit occurs. Frequency increases with age, predisposing factors being atheroma and hypertension. Onset is sudden, usually with loss of consciousness accompanied by gross neurological deficit. Immediate mortality is high. Treatment of those who survive involves correction of risk factors such as hypertension, careful nursing, and physiotherapy. Permanent neurological damage is usual.

Dental Significance

Paralysis and sensory loss may involve the face and mouth, in which case advice and assistance with oral hygiene is required. Wherever possible the natural dentition should be preserved.

IRRITABLE BOWEL SYNDROME (Spastic Colon)

This syndrome is characterized by abdominal pain, altered bowel habit, and flatulence and is the commonest cause of patient referral to gastroenterological clinics.

The symptoms result from disordered muscular function of the bowel, in particular the colon, in the absence of disease. The cause is unknown but is thought to relate to the highly refined foods which constitute western diets.

It is important to exclude organic disease and to reassure the patient to this effect.

Treatment consists of increasing roughage in the diet with bran or other forms of fibre and by the use of smooth muscle relaxants. Response to treatment is unpredictable and often very limited.

Dental Significance

None.

ISCHAEMIC COLITIS, **see** COLITIS

J

JACKSONIAN ATTACKS, see EPILEPSY.

JAUNDICE, see BILIARY DISEASE and LIVER DISEASE.

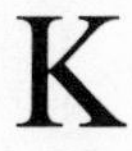

KALA AZAR, see LEISHMANIASIS.

CO-ARCTATION OF THE AORTA

Co-arctation results from a developmental abnormality of the aortic arch. Diagnostic features are high arterial pressures in the upper limbs with lower pressure and delayed pulses in the lower limbs. The important associations are arterial hypertension resulting in cerebral arterial lesions and aortic valve disease. Treatment is surgical correction, without which the average age of death is 35 years.

Dental Significance

Antibiotic cover should be given for all procedures likely to cause a bacteraemia (see HEART DISEASE (Infective), SUBACUTE BACTERIAL ENDOCARDITIS). General anaesthetics should be avoided, and if essential, administered in hospital.

KLINEFELTER'S SYNDROME

This is a variety of male hypogonadism characterized by one or more extra X chromosomes. The condition presents at puberty with gynaecomastia, poor development of secondary sexual characteristics, small testes, and eunuchoidal habitus with disproportionately long legs in relation to the trunk. Intellectual impairment of variable degrees is seen.

Dental Significance

None.

L

LARYNGITIS

Acute infective laryngitis is usually a complication of a cold, influenza, measles, or whooping cough. Besides loss of voice there is usually a dry cough and in children there may be laryngeal oedema and partial respiratory obstruction. Laryngeal oedema can also result from the inhalation of irritants such as steam, chemicals, or regurgitated gastric acid.

Treatment of simple laryngitis consists of resting vocal cords as much as possible and avoiding smoking. Inhalations of **tinct. benz. co.** (friar's balsam), 5 ml to 0.5 litre of boiling water, are usually helpful. Laryngeal oedema requires treatment with **cortisone**, either carried in an aerosol and inhaled such as **betamethasone** (*Becotide*$_{\mathrm{GB}}$) or given systemically. Rarely tracheostomy is required.

Dental Significance

Dental treatment should be postponed for patients suffering from laryngitis, and general anaesthetics avoided.

If, during the course of a general anaesthetic, a patient regurgitates gastric fluid and inhales some, 100 mg of intravenous **hydrocortisone** (*Efcortelan*$_{\mathrm{GB}}$) should be given immediately and the anaesthetic abandoned. Because delayed pulmonary complications can arise following such an event, the patient's doctor should be informed and the patient told to report to him next day.

LAURENCE–MOON–BIEDL SYNDROME

This rare familial disorder is characterized by hypogonadism, dwarfism, obesity, mental deficiency, polydactyly, and retinitis pigmentosa.

Dental Significance

None.

LEGIONNAIRES' DISEASE

An explosive outbreak of fever and pneumonia at an American Legion convention in Philadelphia in 1976 led to the recognition of a previously undescribed group of organisms, *Legionella pneumophila*. Since this time outbreaks and sporadic cases have been described worldwide. Symptoms consist of anorexia, headache, myalgia, and fever, associated with diarrhoea, pleurisy, rigors, and confusion. Mortality rate is about 10 per cent. Treatment consists of rehydration, oxygen, and antibiotics, the most widely used being **erythromycin** (*Erythrocin*$_{\mathrm{GB,US}}$) 2–4 g daily. Respiratory support may be necessary.

Dental Significance

Though there is no evidence of direct person-to-person infection, the disease is thought to be spread by aerosol inhalation and possibly ingestion. A dentist who learns that he has treated a patient suffering from the condition, should warn waiting-room contacts and patients who have been treated in the surgery immediately after.

L

LEISHMANIASIS

This disease results from infection by protozoa of the genus *Leishmania.* Infection may be generalized as with *L. donovani* giving rise to visceral Leishmaniasis or kala-azar. This has a long incubation period and runs a chronic course with remittent fever, leucopenia, and hepatosplenomegaly. Localized infection results from infestation by *L. tropica* causing skin involvement, (the oriental sore), or skin and mucous membrane involvement as seen in mucocutaneous leishmaniasis caused by *L. brasiliensis.*

The parasites are all transmitted to man by a species of the sand-fly *Phlebotomas*. **Antimonial drugs** are the basis of specific treatment.

Dental Significance

In mucocutaneous leishmaniasis chronic destructive ulcers are found in the mouth and pharynx associated with enlarged cervical lymph glands. To confirm the diagnosis smears or ulcer biopsies are examined for intracellular leishman bodies.

LEPROSY (Hansen's Disease)

Leprosy is a specific chronic granulomatous disease caused by *Mycobacterium leprae.* It affects the skin, mucosa of the upper respiratory tract, and peripheral nerves causing neuropathic ulceraton and muscular atrophy.

It occurs worldwide but predominantly in the tropics. It is not very contagious and the mode of transmission remains poorly understood. Prolonged exposure seems necessary and spread is more likely in crowded conditions with poor hygiene. About 200 new cases are reported each year in the USA and about 20 to 30 in GB, almost all in immigrants. Leprosy transmission has not been recorded in England for over 50 years.

Two tissue responses occur:

(1) tuberculoid leprosy with granuloma formation, lymphocyte infiltration, and scanty bacilli;
(2) lepromatous leprosy, a destructive lesion teeming with bacilli.

Treatment is with **dapsone** (*Dapsone*$_{US}$) for at least 2 years in tuberculoid leprosy and 4 years in lepromatous leprosy.

Dental Significance

Lepromatous nodules may occur on the lips, tongue, and palate, and atrophy of the anterior maxilla may cause loosening of the upper incisors. Involvement of peripheral nerves of the mouth will cause numbness in areas supplied.

LEPTOSPIROSIS

This condition is caused by a Gram-negative aerobic spirochaete, *Leptospira icterohaemorrhagica*, whose hosts are man, rat, dog, and cattle, and *L. canicola*, whose hosts are man, dogs, and pigs. Infection is sporadic, classically described in sewage workers and situations where rats occur, but most commonly associated with farming environments. The incidence of the disease is low in the UK. Infection results from environmental contamination by host's urine or by direct contact such as handling infected carcases.

Clinical presentation may be as a pyrexial illness, an enteric illness, nephritis, aseptic meningitis, or as Weil's syndrome. The incubation period is 7–14 days, the illness lasting 2–14 days.

Onset is often sudden with fever, chills, or rigors. There may be headaches, myalgia, arthralgia, and often severe prostration. Renal involvement is common but usually minor; less frequently jaundice and renal failure herald a much more serious form of the disease (Weil's disease). Haemorrhage may be petechial, subconjunctival, or massive bleeding with malaena. Haematemesis, haemoptyses, and ecchymoses occur. Minor pulmonary involvement is common and myocarditis with dysrhythmias occurs.

Mortality is generally about 10 per cent, recovery usually being complete in those who survive. Treatment is with antibiotics, **penicillin** in high dosage being the drug of choice, together with supportive measures for symptoms and complications.

Dental Significance

None.

LEUCOPENIA, see AGRANULOCYTOSIS.

LEUKAEMIA, see LYMPHOPROLIFERATIVE DISORDERS and MYELOPROLIFERATIVE DISORDERS.

LEUKOPLAKIA

Leukoplakia is a negative diagnosis. It is defined by WHO as a white patch which cannot be characterized as other disease. The white patches of the condition are found on the gums, tongue, and cheek and are due to thickening and hyperkeratinization of the mucous membrane. The differential diagnosis from plaque or atrophic-type lichen planus may not be easy. The condition causes little discomfort, and treatment consists of prohibiting smoking, avoiding hot spiced food and concentrated alcohol.

The problem of leukoplakia is its predisposition to malignant change which appears to be greater when it occurs in certain sites in the mouth and when it is associated with candida infection.

Dental Significance

Opinions differ on the pre-cancerous nature of the condition. The association with malignancy may not be close, but, because early detection of it is of such importance, the general practitioner is wise to obtain the opinion of a specialist in all cases of leukoplakia occurring in sites where squamous cell carcinomas of the mouth are found, such as the floor of the mouth and the sides of the tongue.

LICE INFESTATION

The body louse (*Pediculus humanus corporis*), the head louse (*P. humanus capitis*), and the crab louse (*Phthirus pubis*) are obligatory parasites of man.

The louse has a flat segmented body with six legs. The female lays up to five eggs (nits) a day, which adhere to hair and hatch in about 8 days. The nymphs mature in 14 days and live 4–6 weeks. Lice take two blood meals daily, the bite causing considerable irritation. The body louse attaches to body hair and migrates to clothing where it can survive about a day, or if conditions are cold, up to a week. The head louse attaches to scalp hair. Spread occurs during close contact. Relapsing fever (*Borrelia recurrentis*), typhus, and trench fever may be transmitted by lice.

The crab louse attaches to groin and pubic hair and does not usually transmit disease.

Treatment is with **gamma-benzene hexachloride** or **malathion** in shampoo or lotion (*Derbac*$_{GB}$, *Esoderm*$_{GB}$, *Lorexane*$_{GB}$).

Dental Significance

Head-to-head and body-to body contact, or infected clothes, are the usual means of spread, so a dentist is unlikely to pick up the infection from a patient. However if a head looks as if it might be infected close contact with the patient's hair is best avoided.

LICHEN PLANUS

The lesions of this condition appear on the skin as purplish flat patches, and in the mouth as white areas which vary from milk-curd tracery to white plaques and erosions. The condition is more common over the age of 50 and oral and skin lesions occur separately. The cause is unknown.

The main symptom of the skin rash is irritation, while in the mouth the lesions are usually symptom-free unless of the erosive type.

The condition generally resolves on its own, but, if causing discomfort, topical applications of steroids are helpful. On the skin 1 per cent **hydrocortisone** ointment should be applied to the patches, while in the mouth **triamcinolone** dental paste (*Adcortyl*$_{GB}$, *Kenalog*$_{US}$) in orobase should be smeared on, or the areas sprayed with **betamethasone** (*Becotide*$_{GB}$) from an inhaler four times a day after meals.

Dental Significance

Malignant change has occasionally occurred in lichen planus of the erosive or atrophic type, and the dentist should carefully note the character and distribution of the condition and reassess at each visit.

LISTERIA

This condition is caused by a Gram-positive bacillus found worldwide which infects a wide range of animals. In humans, infection is most commonly intrauterine, the mother having a febrile illness and the baby often premature and dying usually soon after birth. Children may have a septicaemic illness with meningitis. In adults an oculoglandular form is seen with pneumonia and occasionally meningitis.

Penicillin is the treatment of choice. Prognosis is good in the adult form but poor in the infant form unless diagnosis is made early.

Dental Significance

None.

LIVER DISEASE

HEPATITIS

This is a diffuse inflammation of the liver which may result from toxins, drugs, or infection. Viral hepatitis is the most common cause and may be subdivided into three main groups.

HEPATITIS A

The virus is transmitted by faecal/oral means though blood spread can occur. It is a disease of poor sanitation, overcrowding, and institutions, especially those for the mentally defective.

It is seen commonly in Third World countries, particularly amongst those travelling to such parts of the world. The virus is present in the blood several days before the liver function tests become abnormal, and disappears with the development of jaundice. The disease is usually self-limiting over a period of weeks though chronic liver disease occasionally results. Serological techniques are now available to confirm infection with the A virus. When travelling abroad to high-risk areas a substantial measure of immunity, lasting 2–3 months, can be obtained by an injection of immune globulin prior to departure. It should not be given within 2 weeks of any live vaccine.

HEPATITIS B

Transmission is almost exclusively parenterally, though recent studies have demonstrated faecal/oral transmission. Whole blood or blood fractions passed at transfusions, via surgical or dental instruments, tattoo needles, or syringe needles are the commonest routes of infection. However, the virus is found in semen, saliva, and urine. The disease is commonest in drug addicts, homosexuals, mentally defectives, and those repeatedly exposed to blood products. The presence of the infection can be confirmed by demonstration of the Australia antigen (Hb_sAg) in serum. This is important, not only in the diagnosis, but also in judging prognosis. In the majority of people the virus is cleared from the blood during recovery following acute illness. In a proportion the virus persists and often this persistence is associated with the development of chronic liver disease. These people are a continuous hazard to others as they are potentially infectious.

HEPATITIS NON-A AND NON-B

This group is probably a heterogeneous group where neither markers for virus A or virus B are found. It is seen most commonly in those people who develop hepatitis following a transfusion, and in haemophiliacs.

Dental Significance

In patients with active hepatitis dental treatment should be postponed until convalescent serological tests reveal the type of virus and whether the patient may still be infective.

HEPATITIS A

Type A hepatitis presents few risks special to the dental surgery. The virus disappears from the blood soon after the arrival of jaundice and has not been demonstrated in the saliva.

HEPATITIS B (formerly known as Australian antigen positive)

In addition to those with active hepatitis, approximately 1 in 1000 of the population of the UK are seriologically Hb_sAg-positive, many having no history of the clinical disease. Of these, 1 in 5 are Hb_eAg-positive and their blood and saliva highly infective. A high proportion of them are to be found among those brought up in developing countries, amongst drug addicts and homosexuals, mongols, and other mentally subnormal cared for in institutions, those with chronic liver disease, haemophiliacs, and those on renal dialysis.

Where possible, dental treatment of patients falling into these categories should be delayed for serological assessments. Those who are Hb_sAg- and Hb_eAg-positive are high-risk patients and should be treated in hospital dental units with special facilities. Those who are Hb_sAg-positive but anti-Hb_e are lesser-risk patients and routine dentistry can be carried out in general practice provided special precautions are taken. These include:

(1) face-masks, gloves, and glasses worn by dentist and assistant;
(2) incineration of contaminated material and disposable instruments after use;
(3) efficient autoclave or dry heat sterilization of all instruments;
(4) work surfaces wiped down with disinfectant containing 1 per cent free chlorine or 2 per cent glutaraldehyde;
(5) impressions to be taken in silicone and immersed in 2 per cent glutaraldehyde for 16 hours before being sent to technicians.

Procedure following accidental inoculation

The blood of patients with active hepatitis and carriers of the disease contains the living virus and will produce the disease if inoculated into another person who is not immune. Modern research indicates that as little as 0.0001 ml of blood from a patient who is Hb_eAg-positive is all that is required, while 1.0 ml of anti-Hb_eAg blood would probably be safe. The virus can also gain entry through an open cut or blood getting in the eyes. The saliva also contains the virus but to lesser extent, and spread by aerosol spray is unlikely. Most dentists cut or pierce their hands from time to time when working on a patient, and if the instrument has been contaminated with blood or saliva they are at risk. When this occurs the dentist is advised to make a careful assessment of the risk through questioning the patient and, if he considers it significant, explain the situation and request the patient has a blood test. The nearest laboratory with facilities for this should be contacted by phone and either arrangements made for the patient to visit immediately or a blood sample taken from the patient in the surgery there and then. This is more efficient and less irksome, and only requires the ability of venepuncture and a few sterile syringes, needles, and specimen bottles which a local pathology laboratory will usually let you have. The procedure is as follows.

(1) With the patient's permission, withdraw 5 ml of venous blood and put it in the specimen bottle avoiding contamination.
(2) Cork the bottle securely (the blood will clot in the bottle but this is anticipated), and label with details of patient and investigation required. Seal bottle in a polythene bag and label bag with sticker saying 'DANGER OF INFECTION' or 'HEPATITIS RISK'. Put needle and syringe in another plastic bag and arrange for them to be incinerated as soon as possible.
(3) Arrange for the specimen to reach the laboratory as soon as possible requesting a result in 36 hours, and if positive appropriate treatment.
(4) Sterilize instruments and disinfect work surfaces and impressions as suggested.

Speed of action is important; the chances of suppressing an attack of hepatitis are much better if hyperimmune gamma-globulin is given within 48 hours. Not only is the dentist at risk when dealing with an infected patient but outbreaks have been traced to dentists carrying the virus. Cuts on the hands should always be covered with waterproof dressings.

Viral hepatitis can have fatal consequences. It is the duty of all dentists to maintain high standards of sterilization and asepsis. Recently a vaccine to offer protection against hepatitis B has been produced. It is undergoing assessment at the time of writing.

CIRRHOSIS

Cirrhosis is a histological diagnosis based on the development of fibrosis in the liver following parenchymal damage. Aetiological classification:

(1) *Cryptogenic*–Commonly no cause for cirrhosis is found.
(2) *Cirrhosis* following chronic active hepatitis.
(3) *Alcoholic cirrhosis.*
(4) *Hepatolenticular degeneration* (Wilson's disease). This is a rare congenital disorder of copper metabolism inherited as an autosomal recessive. The features of the disease result from the deposition of copper mainly in the brain, liver, and kidney due to the deficiency of the copper-carrying protein caeruloplasmin. Damage to the basal ganglia and hepatic cirrhosis result. The importance of the diagnosis is that it is treatable with **penicillamine**.
(5) *Haemochromatosis.* This is cirrhosis due to massive iron accumulation in the liver, due either to a primary abnormality of iron handling by the body or secondary to multiple blood transfusions. Clinical features are those of cirrhosis together with slate grey discoloration of the skin, testicular atrophy, diabetes mellitus, arthropathy, and cardiac failure.

    Diagnosis depends on demonstrating abnormally high serum iron levels and typical biopsy changes.

    Treatment consists of regular venesection and iron chelating agents together with supportive treatment of the complications.
(6) *Immunological liver disease–primary biliary cirrhosis.*

Clinical features of cirrhosis There may be no symptoms or signs in well compensated disease. When symptoms occur they are often vague, dyspepsia, malaise, or tiredness. As the cirrhosis progresses features of liver failure occur: jaundice, ascites, mental deterioration, confusion, and coma. Haematemesis may occur from bleeding varices.

Diagnosis is confirmed by liver biopsy. Management consists of removing the cause where possible and supportive measures for the complications. Prognosis is very variable but the 5-year survival is approximately 5 per cent, death resulting from liver failure, haemorrhage, or hepatoma. Great care should always be taken before the use of any drugs in cirrhotic patients because many are metabolized in the liver and some are hepatotoxic. Cirrhotic patients are particularly sensitive to the effects of sedatives and analgesics.

Dental Significance

An unpleasant smell (foetor hepaticus) is often noticeable in the breath of patients suffering from cirrhosis. Symptomless enlargement of the parotid glands has been reported.

Routine dentistry can be undertaken but a reduced synthesis of blood clotting factors often leads to increased haemorrhage following extractions. **Lignocaine** should be used sparingly not more than 4 ml of 0.2 per cent solution at a visit. **Aspirin** and **paracetamol** should be prescribed with caution and narcotic analgesics avoided. All hypnotics and sedatives can precipitate coma and **diazepam** (*Valium*$_{\text{GB,US}}$) should be used in reduced dosage.

Penicillin is safe to prescribe but **chloramphenicol, erythromycin estolate** (*Ilisone*$_{\text{GB,US}}$) **fusidic acid,** and **talampicillin** (*Talpen*$_{\text{GB}}$) are hepatotoxic.

General anaesthetics should be administered in hospital, and halothane avoided as an anaesthetic agent.

LOEFFLER'S SYNDROME

This is a heterogeneous group of lung disorders associated with eosinophilia in the peripheral blood. There are three main types. In all there is abnormal radiological shadowing on the chest X-ray.

(1) Pulmonary infiltration with eosinophilia but without asthma.

This may result from reaction to parasites such as ascaris, to pollens, or to drugs. Symptoms are a cough and sometimes fever and malaise.

(2) Asthma with eosinophilia.

Although eosinophilia is common in asthma, lung shadowing is not, and, when present, is most commonly due to added infection with *Aspergillus fumigatus*, which causes a hypersensitivity reaction.

(3) Polyarteritis nodosum.

This involves the lung in a third of cases, 50 per cent of whom have eosinophilia and asthma.

Dental Significance

Asthma when present demands the considerations described under asthma.

LUPUS ERYTHEMATOSUS

This multisystem disorder occurs predominantly in young women and is characterized by many non-organ-specific antibodies. As might be expected clinical features are protean and depend on the particular system most affected. They include the characteristic facial 'butterfly' rash, discoid skin lesions, Raynaud's phenomenon, arthritis, pleurisy, pericarditis, psychoses, and nephritis.

Laboratory findings include a normochromic anaemia, positive direct Coombs test, leucopenia, and thrombocytopenia.

The diagnosis is made clinically but supported by the presence of LE cells and anti-nuclear antibodies, and confirmed by antibodies to double-stranded DNA.

Treatment is largely symptomatic and supportive. Steroids, anti-malarials and immunosuppressive drugs have been beneficial in some patients.

Dental Significance

Erythematous patches may be found on the buccal mucosa and gingivae, frequently bilateral, like the butterfly rash on the face. When the disease is widespread (systemic lupus erythematosus) anaemia, leucopenia and thrombocytopenia should be taken into account and extractions carried out under antibiotic cover, anticipating increased post-extraction haemorrhage.

Previous steroid treatment may have depressed the adrenals (see ADRENAL INSUFFICIENCY).

General anaesthetics should be avoided where cardiac and pulmonary complications exist.

LUPUS VULGARIS

This is tuberculous skin involvement usually seen in children, affecting predominantly the face and neck. The skin is scaly, red with telangiectases and the classical 'apple jelly' appearance of individual tubercles when blood is expressed from the lesion with a glass slide. The lesion develops slowly; scarring follows resolution. The bacillus is somewhat attenuated in the skin so **isoniazid** 100 mg three times daily for 6–12 months usually is adequate for curative treatment.

Dental Significance

Lesions in the mouth have been reported, but would resolve with systemic treatment given for the skin.

LYMPHOMA, see **LYMPHOPROLIFERATIVE DISEASE.**

LYMPHOPROLIFERATIVE DISORDERS

Disorders arising from lymphatic tissue.

LEUKAEMIAS

(1) ACUTE LYMPHOBLASTIC LEUKAEMIA

Bone marrow and blood are infiltrated by the most primitive form of lymphoid cell, the lymphoblast. It is more common in children than adults. Aetiological factors include virus infection and irradiation. The clinical features are anaemia, bleeding, and infection.

Treatment with **prednisolone** and **vincristine** (*Oncovin*$_{GB,US}$) leads to complete remission in 95 per cent, further treatment being required to maintain the remission.

(2) CHRONIC LYMPHATIC LEUKAEMIA

This is a malignant proliferation of lymphocytes, more common in men than women and commoner in the elderly. Fifteen per cent of patients are diagnosed on a routine blood count. Clinical features include lymphadenopathy, malaise, anaemia, and splenomegaly. Infection is common due to failure of antibody formation and affects particularly the respiratory system and skin. Haemolytic anaemia and skin infiltration are other complications. The condition does not lead to acute leukaemia.

No treatment is indicated in the absence of symptoms. When required, cytotoxic treatment is with **chlorambucil** (*Leukeran*$_{GB,US}$) or **cyclophosphamide** (*Endoxana*$_{GB}$, *Cytoxan*$_{US}$).

Corticosteroids are used for thrombocytopenia and haemolytic anaemia and radiotherapy for glandular masses. Mean survival is 5 years, with 15 per cent survival to 10 years.

Dental Significance

A third of cases of acute lymphatic leukaemia have oral symptoms from the start and may attend for dental advice before the disease has been diagnosed. In chronic lymphocytic leukaemia oral manifestations tend to occur later.

There is painful swelling of the gingivae associated with infection, bleeding, and sloughing of the overlying mucosa. Large ragged ulcers may occur in the mouth and, as a result of the disease or its treatment with immunosuppressants, secondary infection with bacteria or monilia is common.

Dentists should be alert to the possibility of acute lymphatic leukaemia in the face of painful gingivitis in the young, and appreciate that the white count may be normal and the examination of a blood film necessary to confirm the diagnosis. In established cases every assistance should be given to improve oral hygiene and control secondary infection. Mouthwashes and interdental irrigation with **chlorhexidine** 0.2 per cent (*Corsodyl*$_{GB}$) should be instituted, and candida infection controlled with four-times-daily use of fungicides, such as **nystatin** (*Nystatin mixture*$_{GB}$, *Mycostatin oral suspension*$_{US}$), **amphotericin** lozenges (*Fungilin*$_{GB}$), **miconazole,** or **ketoconazole**.

A viscous mouthwash containing 2 per cent **lignocaine** or **benzocaine** lozenges 10 mg may be required to ease the discomfort of eating. The prescription of antibiotics should be made in consultation with the physician in charge of treatment.

LYMPHOMAS

(1) HODGKIN'S DISEASE

This is a primary disease of lymphoreticular tissue of unknown aetiology, with peak incidence at 25 and 70 years, being commoner in men.

Clinical features are painless glandular enlargement, hepatosplenomegaly, and bone involvement. Symptoms include prurutis, fever, weakness, malaise, weight loss, and anaemia.

Liver involvement leads to jaundice and ascites. Pleural effusions, spinal cord compression, gastrointestinal and skin involvement occur.

Diagnosis depends on biopsy histology. Radiotherapy is the most effective treatment for localized disease. When generalized, chemotherapy is used.

The following group of drugs are used, and are sometimes known as MVPP regime:

(a) nitrogen mustard: **mustine, chlorambucil** (*Leukeran*$_{GB,US}$) or **cyclophosphamide** (*Endoxana*$_{GB}$, *Cytoxan*$_{US}$);
(b) vinca alkaloids: **vincristine** (*Oncovin*$_{GB,US}$) and **vinblastine** (*Velbe*$_{GB}$, *Velban*$_{US}$);
(c) **procarbazine** (*Natulan*$_{GB}$, *Matulane*$_{US}$);
(d) **prednisolone.**

Overall prognosis is good; 80 per cent of patients go into complete remission and 41 per cent are free of disease at 6 years.

Dental Significance

Oral manifestations of Hodgkin's disease are uncommon, and dental problems stem from drugs used in its treatment. Reduced resistance to infection must be expected. Candida infection of the mouth may be controlled with four-times-daily use of oral fungicides, such as **nystatin** (*Nystatin mixture*$_{GB}$, *Mycostatin oral suspension*$_{US}$) or **amphotericin** lozenges (*Fungilin*$_{GB}$). Antibiotic cover should be given if extractions are required, and a reduced platelet count may lead to some post-extraction haemorrhage. Previous treatment with steroids should be taken into account (see ADRENAL INSUFFICIENCY). General anaesthetics should be given in hospital.

NON-HODGKIN'S LYMPHOMAS

There are many similarities between Hodgkin's disease and other lymphomas. Clinical presentation and principles of treatment are the same.

Dental Significance

As for Hodgkin's disease.

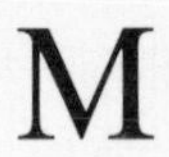

MACROGLOBULINAEMIA (Waldenström macroglobulinaemia)

This is a group of diseases characterized by the presence in the serum of high concentrations of macroglobulin (IgM). It occurs either in isolation or as part of a lymphoproliferative disorder. Clinical features result from hyperviscosity of the blood and include cardiac failure, a bleeding tendency, and retinopathy.

Plasmapheresis may be life-saving, while specific treatment is indicated where lymphoproliferative disease is present.

Dental Significance

Bleeding gums and increased post-extraction haemorrhage are the main oral problems of the condition.

The degree of cardiac failure must be considered when dental treatment is required.

MALARIA

This is probably the most widespread disease of developing countries, caused by the protozoan *Plasmodium*. Four species exist: *P. falciparum, P. vivax, P. malariae,* and *P. ovale.* Transmission is by an anopheles mosquito.

Falciparum malaria may be fatal if treatment is delayed, and it is of the greatest importance to consider the diagnosis in any sick person who has returned from an endemic area in the previous 6 months. The clinical features of the different types are:

(1) MALIGNANT TERTIAN MALARIA (*P. FALCIPARUM*)

This has a variable presentation, which includes headaches, malaise, nausea, vomiting, joint pains, and fever. Few signs are found and deterioration may be dramatic with drowsiness leading to coma, convulsions, and death in 24 hours. Renal failure, hyperpyrexia, and massive haemolysis (black water fever) are other features sometimes seen.

(2) BENIGN TERTIAN (*P. VIVAX*) AND OVALE MALARIA (*P. OVALE*)

Fever is the major feature occurring every second day. Splenomegaly and anaemia occur but serious complications are rare.

(3) QUARTAN MALARIA (*P. MALARIAE*)

This is similar to benign tertian but fever occurs every 3 days and nephrotic syndrome may occur. Diagnosis depends on identifying the parasite in the blood film.

Chloroquine (*Avloclor*$_{GB}$, *Aralen*$_{US}$) cures falciparum malaria without relapse if started in time, because there is no hepatic phase to its life cycle. Treatment of *P. vivax* and *P. ovale* requires additional treatment with **8–aminoquinolone** in order to eradicate the hepatic phase. If uneradicated, relapse of the disease may take place and continue intermittently for 2 or 3 years.

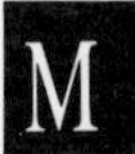

Resistance is increasingly common in south-east Asia, South America and Africa. **Quinine** is the treatment of choice where **chloroquine** resistance is suspected.

Prophylaxis should be taken for a week before entering an endemic area and a month after leaving. One of the following drugs should be used:

proquanil (*Paludrine*$_{GB}$)	100 mg daily
pyrimethamine (*Daraprim*$_{GB,US}$)	50 mg weekly
chloroquine (*Avloclor*$_{GB}$ *Aralen*$_{US}$)	300 mg weekly

Dental Significance

None. There is no danger of the infection being passed on to the dentist or staff.

MALLORY-WEISS SYNDROME

Gastrointestinal haemorrhage occurs in this syndrome due to laceration of the mucosa at the lower end of the oesophagus following vomiting or retching.

Dental Significance

None.

MEASLES (Morbilli)

This highly infectious fever is caused by a virus and has an incubation period of 10–14 days.

The first manifestations are those of a severe cold with fever, conjunctivitis, and sometimes photophobia. The mucosa of the mouth is inflamed and small white Koplik spots are usually visible on the buccal mucosa opposite the molar teeth. The pink/red macular rash appears on the fourth day behind the ears, and spreads to the face and trunk.

The common complications are otitis media and broncho-pneumonia, while a rare but serious one is encephalitis.

The virus is not sensitive to antibiotics but **penicillin V** 250 mg four times daily is given during the acute stage to prevent secondary bacterial infection. Active immunity is obtained by two injections of vaccine but is not given below 9 months of age.

Dental Significance

The disease is spread by droplet infection, a child being most infectious during the first 5 days. Any contacts in the surgery or waiting room should be warned so they may obtain passive immunity with gamma-globulin. Complete suppression may be obtained with a large dose given within 5 days of contact, while a small dose mitigates the condition which still confers active immunity. If measles is severe during early childhood a band of poor enamel may be seen on the teeth when they erupt.

MENIÈRE'S DISEASE

This is a chronic disease of the labyrinth characterized by extremely unpleasant attacks of vertigo associated with tinnitus and progressive deafness. Attacks come on suddenly commencing with buzzing, intense vertigo, nausea, and vomiting with cerebellar signs on the side of the lesion. Attacks usually last 15 minutes to an hour but may last considerably longer.

Treatment is with sedatives and antihistamines such as **dimenhydrinate** (*Dramamine*$_{GB,US}$) 50–100 mg three to six times daily, or **prochlorperazine** (*Stemetil*$_{GB}$, *Compazine*$_{US}$) 5–25 mg as required up to a maximum of 30 mg in 24 hours. Salt-free diet is said to be beneficial. Surgery is required when medical treatment fails.

Dental Significance

Patients generally dislike being placed supine in the dental chair, and treatment in the upright or semi-prone position is more comfortable for them.

METHAEMOGLOBINAEMIA

This abnormal haemoglobin results either from drug interaction such as with phenacetin and sulphonamides, or with industrial poisons such as dinitrobenzene and aniline dyes. A rare congenital form exists. Cyanosis is the striking clinical feature often in the absence of other symptoms. Treatment involves removal of the cause and large doses of **ascorbic acid.**

Dental Significance

None.

MIGRAINE

The presenting symptom is severe headache, accompanied by anorexia, nausea, and vomiting which may last a few hours or 1–2 days. It is usually preceded by a visual aura and thought to result from an initial arterial constriction followed by vasodilatation. The attacks vary in frequency and may be precipitated by a variety of factors such as anxiety, hormones, various foods, or starvation.

Treatment of an attack is with analgesics, usually **aspirin** or **paracetamol**, combined with antinauseants such as **metoclopramide** or **buclizine** (*Migravess*$_{\mathrm{GB}}$, *Paramax*$_{\mathrm{GB}}$, *Migraleve*$_{\mathrm{GB}}$). **Ergotamine** is often helpful and is best given by inhalation (*Medihaler-ergotamine*$_{\mathrm{GB}}$) to obtain rapid absorption.

Prophylactic drugs which are used include **diazepam** (*Valium*$_{GB,US}$), **propranolol** (*Inderal*$_{GB,US}$), **clonidine** (*Dixarit*$_{GB}$), and **methysergide** (*Deseril*$_{GB}$, *Sansert*$_{US}$).

Dental Significance

Occasionally the pain is experienced in the upper teeth, which can cause dental confusion.

Neither the disease itself not the drugs used in its treatment are a hazard to dental treatment.

MIKULICZ SYNDROME

Enlargement of lacrimal and salivary glands due to lymphoma, lymphocytic anaemia, or sarcoid constitute this syndrome.

Dental Significance

This condition is not to be confused with crops or aphthous ulcers, sometimes called Mikulicz ulcers, which are unconnected with the syndrome.

MONGOLISM, see DOWN'S SYNDROME.

MONILIASIS, see CANDIDA INFECTION.

MUCOVISCIDOSIS, see CYSTIC FIBROSIS.

MULTIPLE SCLEROSIS

The cause of this condition remains a mystery—virus infections, deficiency disorders, and autoimmune reactions having all been postulated but not proved. The essential elements are patches of demyelination which occur at random throughout the nervous system, giving rise to localized motor or sensory loss. It is usual for episodes to be followed by periods of remission which may last several years. In those who contract it in middle age the condition is more steadily progressive. There is no effective treatment but **corticotrophin** (*Acthar*$_{GB,US}$) may be helpful during episodes of demyelination.

Dental Significance

Facial numbness is sometimes an early symptom and one which is reported to the dentist.

A number of sufferers have the impression that dental extractions, or even a local anaesthetic for conservative work, evoke demyelinating episodes. Though this has not been substantiated, it should be given consideration, the extent of dental treatment being otherwise dictated by the patient's condition and prognosis.

MUMPS, see **PAROTITIS.**

MUSCULAR DYSTROPHY

This is a group of genetically determined myopathies.

DUCHENNE MUSCULAR DYSTROPHY

This is a sex-linked recessive disorder almost confined to males, developing between the ages of 1½ and 5 years. All muscles except those of the face are ultimately affected but the proximal lower limb muscles are involved first of all. Cardiac involvement and mental retardations are common. Death occurs before the age of 21.

FACIO-SCAPULO-HUMERAL MUSCULAR DYSTROPHY

The inheritance is dominant and the clinical course very variable in this dystrophy. Childhood development carries a poor prognosis but development is usually in the teens when a benign course is seen. Profound facial weakness with winging of the scapulae later leads to limb muscle involvement.

LIMB GIRDLE DYSTROPHY

This rare autosomal recessive disorder has a variable age of onset and initially affects the pelvic girdle causing difficulty in running and climbing stairs. Later the shoulder girdle is involved and severe disability develops by the 4th and 5th decade.

Other dystrophies include Becker type, which is similar to Duchenne dystrophy but more benign, and Ocular and Oculopharyngeal muscular dystrophy involving extra-ocular and pharyngeal muscles with droopy eyelids, limited eye movements, limb weakness, and dysphagia.

Dental Significance

There can be no hard-and-fast rules about the dental treatment of patients with these distressing conditions. The extent and duration of dentistry must be tailored to that which the patient can tolerate, taking into account their life-expectancy.

Many suffer from difficulty in swallowing, and treatment must be unhurried and backed up with efficient suction and surgery assistance. General anaesthetics are to be avoided.

MYASTHENIA GRAVIS

Pathological fatiguability of muscles is the dominant feature of this rare disorder of neuromuscular junctions. It is seen at all ages, more commonly in women.

Clinical features are muscle weakness of one or more muscle groups, most commonly extra-ocular and facial, but also bulbar, neck, shoulder, and hip muscles. Bulbar and respiratory paralysis may occur. Diagnosis is clinical and confirmed by the response to intravenous **edrophonium chloride** (*Tensilon*$_{GB,US}$).

Treatment is with anticholinergic drugs, **neostigmine bromide** (*Prostigmin*$_{GB,US}$) 15 mg tablets three or four times a day or **pyridostigmine** (*Mestinon*$_{GB,US}$) 60 mg three of four times a day. Intoxication by anticholinergic drugs may lead to a cholinergic crisis, when treatment with assisted ventilation is necessary. **Prednisolone** and immunosuppressive drugs may be valuable in more severe cases. Thymectomy has beneficial results and is now being carried out earlier in the disease.

Dental Significance

Dental treatment should be carried out in the mornings, mouth props and efficient suction being helpful to the patient. **Neostigmine** should be taken by the patient 20 minutes before the start of treatment. Local anaesthetics should be administered with caution and **diazepam** (*Valium*$_{GB,US}$) and **streptomycin** avoided, as they may make the condition worse. General anaesthetics should be avoided, and where essential conducted in hospital.

MYASTHENIC SYNDROME (Eaton Lambert)

This condition resembles myasthenia gravis in so far as muscle fatiguability occurs, but response to neostigmine is poor or absent and reflexes are usually depressed or missing. It is usually associated with oat-cell carcinoma of bronchus.

Dental Significance

Patients with this condition are unlikely to attend for dental treatment.

MYELOFIBROSIS, see MYELOPROLIFERATIVE DISORDERS.

MYELOMA

Multiple myeloma is a malignant disease of plasma cells resulting in production of abnormal immunoglobulins from a single clone of cells. This gives rise to a homogeneous immunoglobulin, a paraprotein, or M protein.

Symptoms result from skeletal destruction causing crush vertebral fractures and bone pain. Disturbance of immunoglobulin leads to infection, and marrow replacement to anaemia and bleeding. Renal failure results from hypercalcaemia and protein deposition in the kidney.

Treatment includes analgesics for pain, the management of complications, anaemia, infection, and renal failure and specific therapy with **melphalan** (*Alkeran*$_{GB,US}$) or **cyclophosphamide** (*Endoxana*$_{GB}$, *Cytoxan*$_{US}$).

Dental Significance

Myelomas may develop in the mandible and give rise to pain, resorption of roots, and loosening of teeth. Radiologically they appear as round translucent areas. Increased susceptibility to infection and haemorrhage are complications of the disease.

MYELOPROLIFERATIVE DISORDERS

Proliferative disorders of the granulocytic, megakaryocytic, and erythroid series are known as the myeloproliferative syndrome.

LEUKAEMIA

ACUTE MYELOGENOUS LEUKAEMIA (AML)

An accumulation of primitive blast cells is seen in this condition. The aetiology is unknown but might possibly be viral. Clinical features are similar to those of acute lymphoblastic leukaemia; symptoms of anaemia; and complications of haemorrhage, infection, and tissue infiltration. It occurs more frequently in the middle-aged and elderly than in the young, and is uncommon in childhood. Treatment involves various chemotherapeutic regimes incorporating **cytarabine** (*Cytosar*$_{\mathrm{GB}}$, *Cytosar-U*$_{\mathrm{US}}$), an inhibitor of DNA synthesis, together with supportive care, treatment of anaemia and haemorrhage, and prompt treatment of infection.

Prior to chemotherapy few survived and 50 per cent died within 2 months. Now, at least half of those developing AML achieve complete remission.

CHRONIC MYELOID LEUKAEMIA

The onset of this disorder is insidious, occurring more commonly in males and usually between the ages of 20 and 60 years.

Clinical features are weakness, fatigue, malaise, loss of weight, and sweating. Splenomegaly and hepatomegaly may cause abdominal discomfort and dyspepsia. Bleeding problems tend to occur later in the disease. Diagnosis is based on a high white cell count, usually greater than 50,000/ml, with myelocytes, metamyelocytes, and occasional blast cells. Platelets are often increased in number, the leucocyte alkaline phosphatase is low, and serum B12 level high.

There is a good response to chemotherapy with **busulphan** (*Myleran*$_{GB,US}$) and remission is easily maintained for 2–3 years. However, sometimes the disease runs a rapid course.

Dental Significance

As with lymphatic leukaemias, oral manifestations are worse in the acute disease and may be the presenting symptom. There is painful swelling of the gingivae associated with infection, bleeding, and sloughing of the overlying mucosa. Large ragged ulcers may occur in the mouth, and as a result of the disease or its treatment with immunosuppressants, secondary infection with bacteria or monilia is common.

Every assistance should be given to improve oral hygiene and control infection. Mouthwashes and interdental irrigation with **chlorhexidine** 0.2 per cent (*Corsodyl*$_{GB}$) should be instituted, and candida infection controlled with four-times-daily use of oral fungicides such as **nystatin** (*Nystatin mixture*$_{GB}$, *Mycostatin oral suspension*$_{US}$), **amphotericin** lozenges (*Fungilin*$_{GB}$), **miconazole,** or **ketoconazole**. If discomfort is severe 2 per cent viscous **lignocaine** or **benzocaine** lozenges will ease the pain of eating. Dentures should only be worn for meals. The prescription of antibiotics must be made in consultation with the physician in charge of treatment.

MYELOFIBROSIS

In this bone marrow disorder fibrous tissue and sometimes new bone is laid down. In its primary form the cause is unknown, but it may occur secondary to toxic damage to the marrow. The blood picture is of a leuco-erythroblastic anaemia with extramedullary haematopoiesis and hepatosplenomegaly.

Onset is insidious in late middle age with fatigue, weaknes, and symptoms due to huge splenomegaly and anaemia. The disease runs a prolonged course, infection being a major complication and cause of death. Average survival is 5 years from the time of diagnosis.

Treatment is supportive, androgenic steroids may be beneficial, splenectomy may be indicated for a very large spleen or hypersplenism.

Dental Significance

Strict attention to oral hygiene and the control of bacterial and fungal infections of the mouth is important (see LEUKAEMIA). Antibiotic cover is essential for extractions.

POLYCYTHAEMIA RUBRA VERA

This chronic myeloproliferative disorder results in excessive production of red cells causing an increased total red cell mass, packed cell volume, and red cell count. The aetiology is unknown. It occurs more commonly in men and in late middle age. Non-specific symptoms include headaches, dizziness, tinnitus, and pruritus. Patients have a plethoric appearance. The main features of the disease result from increased blood viscosity and include venous and arterial thromboses, occasionally haemorrhage, ischaemic heart disease, and cerebral symptoms with signs of ischaemia and infarction. Splenomegaly increases with the duration of the disease. Treatment is by venesection in the acute phase in combination with ^{32}**P** or cytotoxic drugs, **chlorambucil** (*Leukeran*$_{GB,US}$), **cyclophosphamide** (*Endoxana*$_{GB}$, *Cytoxan*$_{US}$), or **busulphan** (*Myleran*$_{GB,US}$). Without treatment mean survival is 2 years; with venesection mean survival is 4 years, while the combination of venesection and ^{32}**P** or cytotoxic treatment increases survival to more than 10 years. Early deaths result from thrombosis or haemorrhage, late deaths from marrow failure or leukaemia.

SECONDARY POLYCYTHAEMIA

As in polycythaemia rubra vera, this condition is associated with increased erythropoietin and an increased red cell mass. It occurs in chronic hypoxic states (i.e. congenital cyanotic heart disease, chronic respiratory failure, and exposure to high altitude). It is also seen in association with certain tumours, renal carcinoma, uterine fibroids, cerebellar haemangioblastomas, and hepatomas.

Dental Significance

The oral mucous membrane is often blue-red in colour with atrophic glossitis and angular cheilitis present.

Post-extraction haemorrhage can be severe, and though blood loss may be beneficial it is better controlled by venesection. When teeth have to be lost they should be extracted one at a time with precautions to arrest bleeding.

THROMBOCYTHAEMIA

Essential haemorrhagic thrombocythaemia may accompany any of the myeloproliferative syndromes. Patients present with haemorrhagic tendencies because the platelets are abnormal in function as well as number. In addition splenomegaly, moderate leucocytosis, and a high leucocyte alkaline phosphatase are seen.

Prognosis is usually good, although late in the disease lethal forms of myeloproliferative disease may develop.

Treatment is with intermittent ^{32}P.

Dental Significance

Bleeding may occur from the gums and submucosal haemorrhages appear on the palate. Extractions should not be undertaken without consultation with the patient's physician.

MYOCARDIAL INFARCTION, see HEART DISEASE (Ischaemic).

MYOCARDITIS

Myocarditis is acute damage to heart muscle due to infection, most commonly viral, or toxic agents. Clinical features are a sinus tachycardia, dysrhythmias, and occasionally heart failure. Pericarditis may be an additional feature especially when the infective agent is Coxsackie B virus. Non-specific abnormalities are seen on the ECG. Treatment is symptomatic and supportive.

Dental Significance

Patients are too ill to attend for dental treatment.

MYOTONIA ATROPHICA, see DYSTROPHIA MYOTONICA.

MYXOEDEMA, see THYROID DISEASE.

N

NEPHRITIS, see RENAL DISEASE.

NEPHROTIC SYNDROME, see RENAL DISEASE.

NEUROFIBROMATOSIS

Neurofibromata are benign tumours of the connective tissue sheath and may arise singly on any nerve. They cause no symptoms unless situated where the nerve lies in a bony canal or is constricted by other structures, in which case neuritis and degeneration of the nerve may occur. Developing within the cranium or spinal canal, symptoms from pressure on adjacent nerves will be evident.

Multiple neurofibromata of cutaneous nerves (von Recklinghausen's disease) usually appear in childhood or adolescence. They are frequently associated with areas of skin pigmentation (café-au-lait spots) and bone and endocrine disorders (Phaeochromocytoma). The tumours form small lumps in the skin varying in size from that of a pea to several centimetres in diameter. In many instances there is a family history of the disorder. There is no treatment other than surgical removal where they are large and unsightly or causing pressure symptoms.

Dental Significance

In a few cases the neurofibromata appear in the mouth.

Loss of sensation over the face, eye, or mouth will result from presure on the trigeminal nerve and facial weakness if the 7th nerve is involved.

The possibility of an endocrine disorder should be borne in mind when planning a general anaesthetic.

NEUROSYPHILIS, see SYPHILIS.

NEUTROPOENIA, see AGRANULOCYTOSIS.

O

O

OBESITY

Although certain pathological conditions can predispose to excess weight (e.g. hypothyroidism, Cushing's disease, and hypothalamic damage), almost invariably no underlying pathology exists. However, simple obesity is seen in families and certain races, and although this may be attributed to environmental influences and eating patterns it seems probable that an abnormality of fat metabolism exists in some obese subjects.

Obesity is common in affluent society the world over, and constitutes one of the greatest health problems in the western world. Life expectancy is greatly reduced, as is reflected in insurance premiums for obesity. Other complications include skeletal damage, an increased tendency to diabetes, and heart disease. Respiratory complications in extreme obesity, psychiatric disturbances, and problems with general anaesthesia and surgery lead to a greatly increased morbidity and mortality rate.

Treatment ranges from dieting to tooth-wiring and bypass gastrointestinal surgery. Response to dieting is often short-lived and usually compliance is poor. Intermaxillary tooth-wiring is effective and safe but weight tends to be regained once wires are removed due to a resumption of excessive calorie intake. Surgery is hazardous except when performed in centres specializing in such procedures and able to provide careful long-term follow-up.

Dental Significance

Gross obesity complicates all dental treatment. Inferior dental nerve blocks are difficult to position accurately and the mass of the cheeks limits access for conservation and surgery.

General anaesthesia is fraught with problems of keeping the airway open if the patient is not intubated, while intubation in itself becomes a more difficult procedure. Wherever possible local anaesthesia should be used, reinforced with conscious sedation techniques when required.

Fenfluramine (*Ponderax*$_{\text{GB}}$, *Pondimin*$_{\text{US}}$) is a drug frequently prescribed in obesity. Patients taking it may complain of a dry mouth. General anaesthetics should be conducted with caution on patients being treated with this drug, as a fatality has been reported.

Before co-operating in tooth-wiring a dentist should carefully assess the patient's dentition to make sure little permanent damage will result, and carry out conservative and periodontal treatment to render the mouth as healthy as possible. To avoid gingival damage the jaws are best fixed by wires or attachments direct-bonded onto the buccal surfaces of the teeth and wired together. Alternatively metal or acrylic cap-splints can be constructed with opposing hooks for wire ligatures. Meticulous instructions to maintain oral hygiene are essential and **chlorhexidine** 0.2 per cent (*Corsodyl*$_{\text{GB}}$) mouthwash well rinsed between the teeth four times daily, is advisable.

OSLER RENDU WEBER SYNDROME see HEREDITARY HAEMORRHAGIC TELANGIECTASIS.

OSTEITIS DEFORMANS (Paget's Disease)

More common in men than in women, the disease is said to be

present in 3 per cent of men over 40, but in most cases is symptomless. Essentially there is abnormal osteoclastic resorption accompanied by disorderly apposition of new bone. The bones affected in order of frequency are the lumbar sacral spine, pelvis, tibia, femur, clavicles, and skull.

Bone pain, osteoarthrosis, and deafness are the usual symptoms. Bending of weight-bearing bones and pathological fracture are common. Sarcoma is luckily rare. The peripheral resistance of the circulation is altered if the disease is widespread and 'high-output' cardiac failure may follow.

There is no cure but **calcitonin** (*Calcitare*$_{GB}$, *Calcimar*$_{US}$) injections of 40–160 units daily are helpful.

Dental Significance

The bones of the jaw are occasionally affected, causing enlargement, spreading of teeth and mental anaesthesia. On the X-ray the lamina dura is missing and the cancellous bone has a ground-glass or cotton-wool appearance. Hypercementosis may be seen on roots of teeth. In the early stages of the disease, characterized by increased vascularity, excessive bleeding follows dental extractions. Later, with bone sclerosis and hypercementosis, extractions become difficult with increased liability to post-operative infection and sequestrae. Enlargement of the dental ridges in the edentulous produces problems with the fit of dentures.

OSTEITIS FIBROSA CYSTICA, see PARATHYROID DISEASE.

OSTEOARTHRITIS

This very common disorder may be primary where the cause is unknown or secondary to trauma infection or inflammation. It may be associated with certain occupations and with obesity. Frequency increases with age. Joints most commonly affected are the knees, hips, distal interphalangeal joints, and the carpo-metacarpal joint of the thumb. However almost any joint may be affected, including the temporomandibular joint. Pain and stiffness are gradual in onset and usually absent at rest. Treatment ranges from simple analgesia to anti-inflammatory agents such as **naproxen** (*Naprosyn*$_{GB,US}$) and **indomethacin** (*Indocin*$_{GB,US}$) and ultimately surgery where hip replacement has provided some of the most dramatically successful results.

Dental Significance

Osteoarthritis of the temporomandibular joint is comparatively uncommon, in the absence of previous trauma. When occurring in the edentulous or those with severe attrition, restoration of correct vertical occlusion is important. Non-steroidal anti-inflammatory drugs such as **naproxen** (*Naprosyn*$_{GB,US}$) 250 mg twice daily may be helpful, but should not be prescribed for those with a history of peptic ulceration.

OSTEOGENESIS IMPERFECTA

In this disease, characterized by a deficiency of the collagen matrix, the bones are fragile and subject to frequent fracture. In some cases the sclerae of the eyes are blue, the skull enlarged horizontally, and hearing impaired through otosclerosis.

There is no treatment but fractures occur less frequently as children grow older.

Dental Significance

Dentagenesis imperfecta, with brown or grey dentine, sometimes accompanies the disease. The density of the bone of the mandible is reduced and lower incisors may be fanned forward by the tongue. Mandibular fracture during extractions has not been reported as a hazard.

Patients with osteogenesis imperfecta are said to be more liable to malignant hyperthermia as a result of general anaesthetics, and these should therefore be conducted in hospital.

OSTEOMALACIA

The same conditions which produce rickets in the young lead to osteomalacia in the adult; namely dietary deficiency of vitamin D, absorption failure, or resistance to its action. It is to be found in the elderly and debilitated, Asian immigrants, and those on anticonvulsant drugs or aluminium hydroxide. It is also associated with renal disease, diseases of the gastrointestinal tract, and chronic liver disease.

The mineral content of the bone is depleted with an increase in cancellous bone and osteoid. Bone pain and proximal muscle weakness are common, and pseudo and pathological fractures occur.

Treatment is with **cholecalciferol** or one of the recently synthesized forms of **vitamin D**, the dosage depending on the aetiology of the condition.

Dental Significance

The teeth are unaffected but the cortical bone of the jaw and the lamina dura are reduced in thickness, with greater liability to fracture. This demands caution when extracting teeth.

OSTEOPETROSIS (Albers-Schönberg's disease)

This rare hereditary disease is characterized by increased thickness of cortical bone at the expense of the medulla.

'Marble bones' and 'celery stick' are terms coined to describe their radiographic appearance. Patients suffer from anaemia, compression of cranial nerves, and pathological fractures.

There is no treatment.

Dental Significance

Abnormal teeth and delayed eruption has been reported when the disease occurs in juveniles. In adults extractions are difficult and should be undertaken with antibiotic cover as a precaution against osteomyelitis.

OSTEOPOROSIS

In this condition, which mainly affects the elderly, there is a general reduction in bone substance, involving both matrix and mineral content. It is seen in women following the menopause but it is likely that at least a third of us are affected by the condition after the age of 60. Immobilization, hyperthyroidism, rheumatoid arthritis, and prolonged steroid administration are predisposing factors. The sequelae are pathological fractures most commonly of the vertebrae, the neck of the femur, or the wrist.

Treatment consists of giving **calcium** (*Sandocal*$_{\mathrm{GB}}$) three times daily to produce a calcium intake of 1–1.5 g per day. Oestrogens in women, and androgens in men, may be helpful.

Dental Significance

The cortical bone of upper and lower jaws is greatly reduced in thickness and bone trabeculae reduced in number. The maxillary antrum is increased in size and dips down between the roots of the molars. Excessive force during dental extractions can cause fracture of the maxillary tuberosity or the mandible.

OTITIS

OTITIS EXTERNA

Inflammation of the external auditory meatus, may be acute and painful when resulting from a boil or furuncle in the ear. More commonly it takes the form of a dermatitis or eczema of the meatal skin.

Treatment of the acute bacterial infection is with systemic wide-spectrum antibiotics such as oral **amoxycillin** (*Amoxil*$_{GB,US}$) 250–500 mg three times daily, while chronic otitis externa is usually treated with topical applications of steroid combined with antimicrobial and fungicidal agents.

OTITIS MEDIA

Inflammation of the middle ear, is more common in children. Below the age of 4 *Haemophilus influenza* is the common infective agent, while later a streptococcus is more usual. Pain is acute and there is danger of perforation of the drum if the infection is not brought under control quickly. When the condition is severe an initial dose of **amoxycillin** (*Amoxil*$_{GB,US}$) should be given by intramuscular injection (125–500 mg according to age) and then 125–500 mg by mouth three times daily. **Trimethoprim** (*Monotrim*$_{GB}$, *Proloprim*$_{US}$) either alone or in combination with **sulphamethoxazole** (*Bactrim*$_{GB}$, *Septrin*$_{GB}$, *Septra*$_{US}$) may also be used in treatment of the condition. Chronic otitis media often requires myringotomy and paracentesis with or without insertion of a grommet tube.

Dental Significance

Patients with pain originating in the ear sometimes present to the dentist thinking it comes from a back tooth. This should be borne in mind if no dental pathology can be found.

P

PAGET'S DISEASE see OSTEITIS DEFORMANS.

PANCREATIC DISEASE

PANCREATITIS

ACUTE PANCREATITIS

This condition presents dramatically with severe abdominal pain of sudden onset accompanied by pallor and often shock. It usually necessitates urgent admission to hospital, where it must be differentiated from other abdominal emergencies and acute myocardial infarction. The main aetiological factors are alcohol and gallstones.

Diagnosis is made clinically and supported by very high serum amylase levels.

Treatment commences with immediate resuscitatory measures. Where the patient is shocked, intravenous fluid replacement, avoidance of oral nutrition, nasogastric suction, and appropriate analgesia are required. Only in the face of real diagnostic doubt is laparotomy indicated. Pancreatitis may be complicated by diabetes, jaundice, pseudocyst formation, tetany, hypotension, and renal failure. Mortality rates in acute pancreatitis are as high as 30 per cent, but those who recover usually do well and few develop relapsing pancreatitis.

RELAPSING PANCREATITIS (ACUTE RELAPSING)

This uncommon condition, characterized by recurrent attacks of acute pancreatitis, leads to progressive pancreatic damage, pancreatic insufficiency, and diabetes.

CHRONIC PANCREATITIS

P

This disorder is characterized by destruction of glandular tissue associated with fibrosis and calcification leading to exocrine and endocrine failure. Unlike acute pancreatitis, biliary disease seems unrelated but chronic alcoholism may be causative in some people. It does not seem to follow acute pancreatitis. Presentation may be purely with central abdominal pain and no pancreatic insufficiency, or with insufficiency and no pain. Frequently both co-exist. Treatment is symptomatic, the constant need for strong painkillers often leading to drug dependency. Insufficiency may be helped by oral **pancreatic enzyme** preparations, and **insulin** may be required to control diabetes.

Dental Significance

Co-existing diabetes must always be considered when treating patients with pancreatic disease (see DIABETES MELLITUS). Oral ulceration and irritation of perioral skin has been reported in those taking **pancreatin** in liquid form.

PARALYSIS AGITANS (PARKINSON'S DISEASE)

This common condition of advancing age results from degeneration of the basal ganglia and substantia nigra.

The clinical features are a 'pill-rolling' tremor of the hands; tremor of the legs, jaw, and head occurring at rest and diminishing with activity. In addition increased muscle tone occurs, giving rise to the characteristic 'lead-pipe' rigidity which may take on a 'cogwheel' character when the tremor is present. Postural abnormalities, akinesia giving a mask-like appearance to the face, slowness in initiating movements, mental deterioration, dribbling, and micturition difficulties are common accompanying features. Parkinson's disease may follow encephalitis and Parkinsonism results from certain drugs (i.e. **phenothiazines**), but in most cases the aetiology is unknown.

Levadopa is the most powerful available form of treatment and is used in combination with **carbidopa** (*Sinemet*$_{GB,US}$) an extracerebral decarboxylase inhibitor or **benserazide** (*Madopar*$_{GB}$).

For mild symptoms, **amantadine** (*Symmetrel*$_{GB,US}$) or anticholinergic drugs such as **benzhexol** (*Artane*$_{GB,US}$) or **orphenadrine** (*Disipal*$_{GB,US}$) are used.

Dental Significance

Tremor may affect the jaw and tongue but does not preclude routine dental treatment. Some difficulty in swallowing is common, and efficient suction is an important adjunct.

Complaints of a dry mouth are frequent with those on treatment with **amantadine** (*Symmetrel*$_{GB,US}$) and **benzhexol** (*Artane*$_{GB,US}$). Providing the condition is mild and uncomplicated by other disease, general anaesthetics may be administered at the surgery. Halothane should be avoided in these patients being treated with **levadopa.**

PARATHYROID DISEASE

HYPERPARATHYROIDISM

Primary hyperparathyroidism is usually the result of hyperplasia, adenoma, or rarely carcinoma of a parathyroid gland. The condition is said to be as common as 1 in 1000 in the UK, and is more frequent in women.

It may present on account of renal stone formation with colic, haematuria, renal infection, and occasionally, if diagnosed late, renal failure. Alternatively it may present with symptoms of hypercalcaemia, anorexia, dyspepsia, weakness, headache, constipation, polyuria, and mental changes. A less common presentation is with symptoms of metabolic bone disease, bone pain, and pathological fractures. Extensive osteolytic bone changes—most commonly seen in the jaws, tibiae, and fingers—are demonstrated radiologically (osteitis fibrosa cystica).

Diagnosis depends on finding a high serum calcium and alkaline phosphatase, a low phosphate, and high parathormone level.

Definitive treatment is surgical removal of the affected gland.

Secondary hyperparathyroidism is the response of the parathyroid glands to a low serum calcium, and is seen predominantly in renal disease and malabsorption. Symptoms are of the underlying cause and also of the resultant metabolic bone disease, skeletal pain, proximal muscle weakness, rickets in children, pseudo and pathological fractures. In contrast to primary hyperparathyroidism the serum calcium is low.

Treatment is the correction where possible of the underlying disorder and administration of **vitamin D**. This needs to be given in large doses in renal disorders.

Tertiary hyperparathyroidism is a pathological extension of secondary hyperparathyroidism when the gland develops autonomous activity leading to a rise in the serum calcium.

Dental Significance

On X-ray there is thinning of the cortical bone, loss of trabeculae and lamina dura, and the appearance of symptomless giant-cell cysts in the bones of the jaw. These only become noticed by the patient if they break through to the surface and present as an epulis.

Not all giant-cell epulides are associated with hyperparathyroidism, but multiple or recurrent ones should alert the dentist to the possibility. Diagnosis is important so that the patient may obtain treatment before irreversible renal damage has occurred.

HYPOPARATHYROIDISM

This can occur spontaneously, but more usually results from surgical removal of the parathyroid glands by design or during thyroidectomy. The level of serum calcium falls and tetany with muscle cramps and epileptic fits may occur. In long-standing hypocalcaemia there is a dry scaly skin, brittle nails, and loss of hair.

Treatment is with **calcium** and **vitamin D** in high doses.

Dental Significance

Hypoparathyroidism in infants will cause enamel hypoplasia but in the adult no changes in teeth or bones are seen.

PARKINSON'S DISEASE, see PARALYSIS AGITANS.

PAROTITIS

PYOGENIC PAROTITIS

This is an ascending infection occurring in the debilitated and those with acute specific fevers. It is prevented by attention to oral hygiene and antibiotics.

EPIDEMIC PAROTITIS (Mumps)

This is a viral disease, spread by saliva contact or droplet infection, with an incubation period of 3–4 weeks. The painful swelling of the parotid glands is usually bilateral and the orifice of Stensen's duct inflamed. In adolescents and adults complications are not infrequent and include orchitis, oophoritis, pancreatitis, and encephalitis. The only treatment is symptomatic.

Mumps vaccine is given as a preventative measure in the USA, together with rubella and measles vaccine. It is not in general use in the UK.

Dental Significance

Children with mumps may be brought to the dentist complaining of pain on eating, and the tender salivary glands need to be distinguished from lymphadenitis resulting from oral infection or tonsillitis. If the condition is suspected, instruments and utensils contaminated with saliva must be carefully sterilized.

PAROXYSMAL TACHYCARDIA, see HEART DISEASE (Dysrhythemia).

PATENT DUCTUS ARTERIOSUS, see HEART DISEASE (Congenital).

PEDICULOSIS, see LICE INFECTION.

PEMPHIGOID

This skin disorder is similar to pemphigus but affects an older age group and may be preceded by urticarial and eczematous reactions. The blisters are large and remain intact longer, being entirely subepidermal. The cause is unknown. Treatment is with systemic steroids.

Dental Significance

As in the skin, the bullae in the mouth remain intact for longer than in pemphigus. They are frequently associated with a painful gingivitis.

Treatment is as for pemphigus.

PEMPHIGUS

This rare condition of middle age begins with ulceration of mouth, conjuctiva, and in women, vulva, leading to crops of bullae ½–1 cm in diameter which rupture easily leaving a raw bleeding area. The bullae occur within the epidermis. Untreated the condition may be fatal. Its cause is unknown.

Treatment is with systemic steroids.

Dental Significance

Oral lesions are said to be present in every case of pemphigus and may precede the skin eruption by as much as a year. Bullae break down rapidly in the mouth and the condition presents as superficial ulcers on the buccal mucosa, lips and palate. Discomfort may be marked.

Topical steroids in the form of **hydrocortisone** pellets (*Corlan*$_{GB}$) 2.5 mg or **triamcinolone** paste (*Adcortyl*$_{GB}$, *Kenalog*$_{US}$) in orobase, four times daily will help, but severe cases require **corticosteroids** systemically.

PEPTIC ULCERATION

Peptic ulcers occur in parts of the gastrointestinal tract where acid and pepsin are secreted, most commonly the stomach and first part of duodenum but occasionally the oesophagus and rarely in a Meckel's diverticulum. They are unusual in children but common in adults, occurring in ten per cent of the population at some stage of their lives. Gastric ulcers occur equally in men and women; duodenal ulcers are three times more common in men. The aetiology remains obscure but acid is an essential ingredient and presumably some defect in the mucosal defence is another.

Pain is the main symptom, usually related to eating and often associated with loss of appetite and nausea.

Modern diagnostic techniques have shown that the traditionally accepted symptomatic differences between gastric and duodenal ulcers do not exist and differentiation can only be made by barium meal or endoscopy.

Major advances in treatment have come with the development of powerful H2 receptor blockers **cimetidine** (*Tagamet*$_{GB,US}$) and **ranitidine** (*Zantac*$_{GB}$) which lower gastric acid production. In addition *De-Nol*, a bismuth preparation, and **carbenoxolone** (*Biogastrone*$_{GB}$) heal ulcers by different mechanisms and are extremely effective in ulcer treatment. The latter causes fluid retention and cannot be used in the elderly and those with heart disease.

More than thirty different antacids are available for symptomatic treatment. Endoscopic examination and biopsy is recommended for all gastric ulcers to exclude carcinoma.

The main complications are haemorrhage, perforation, and pyloric stenosis.

Dental Significance

Aspirin and aspirin-containing analgesics, **diflunisal** (*Dolo-*

bid$_{GB}$), **mefenamic acid** (*Ponstan*$_{GB}$, *Ponstel*$_{US}$) or non-steroidal anti-inflammatory drugs should not be prescribed for patients with peptic ulcers. **Paracetamol** is a safe alternative. For more severe pain **dextropropoxyphene** (*Distalgesic*$_{GB}$, *Darvon-N*$_{US}$) or **dihydrocodeine** (*DF 118*$_{GB}$), may be taken every 4–6 hours.

Delayed gastric emptying may be a feature of the disease and drugs used in its treatment, and it is wise to allow an interval of 6 hours between the last meal and a general anaesthetic.

Diazepam (*Valium*$_{GB,US}$) should be used with caution on those being treated with **cimetidine** (*Tagamet*$_{GB,US}$) as its action is prolonged.

PERICARDITIS

This is inflammation of the pericardium and may be accompanied by a pericardial effusion.

ACUTE PERICARDITIS

This may result from infection, most commonly viral, collagen disorders, chemical and metabolic upsets, e.g. uraemia, myocardial infarction, and trauma.

CHRONIC CONSTRICTIVE PERICARDITIS

This frequently follows previous tuberculosis but in many cases no cause is found. Interference with normal heart function leads to circulatory failure.

Treatment of acute pericarditis depends on the cause, and usually consists of supportive therapy.

Where possible surgery is the treatment of choice in chronic constrictive pericarditis.

Dental Significance

Patients with acute pericarditis are unlikely to attend for dental treatment, and a past history of the condition poses no contra-indications to dentistry unless constrictive pericarditis has developed. In patients with this complication the output of the heart is compromised and general anaesthetics should only be administered in hospital.

PERIODIC FAMILIAL PARALYSIS, see FAMILIAL PERIODIC PARALYSIS.

PERNICIOUS ANAEMIA, see ANAEMIA.

PERTUSSIS (Whooping Cough)

Pertussis is one of the more distressing infectious fevers of childhood, on occasions leading to permanent lung damage and having a mortality rate of 1 per 1000 among infants under 6 months. There is no maternal conferred immunity, and whooping cough vaccine is seldom offered under 6 months and then only accepted by 60 per cent of the population of Great Britain at the present time.

The incubation period is 7–14 days, and the illness starts like a chesty cold from which develop the paroxysms of coughing with the characteristic whoop. Treatment with **erythromycin** renders the child non-infectious but only alleviates the symptoms.

Dental Significance

There are no specific points of dental significance but dentists should bear in mind the infectivity of an untreated child and the chance of passing on the infection to another in waiting room or surgery. Prophylaxis can be obtained by giving **erythromycin** 12.5 mg/kg four times a day for 2 weeks, provided it is started within 6 days of contact.

PETIT MAL, see EPILEPSY.

PEUTZ–JEGHERS SYNDROME

Patchy mucocutaneous pigmentation and adenomatous polyps, predominantly of the small intestine, are the main features of this inherited condition. Symptoms result from the polyps and include bouts of abdominal pain, borborygmi, bleeding, and symptoms of anaemia. Carcinoma is not a complication of this type of polyposis,

Dental Significance

The brown or black patches of pigmentation may occur round the lips and in the mouth.

PHAEOCHROMOCYTOMA, see ADRENAL DISEASE.

PHARYNGITIS

Pharyngitis or sore throat is seldom a disease in itself but a prodromal symptom of a cold, influenza, or one of the infectious fevers of childhood. The causative agent is frequently a virus and initial treatment with antibiotics not warranted unless accompanying lymphangitis. An exception is acute epiglottitis, which is more prevalent below the age of 6 and is due to *Haemophilus influenzae* Type B. Urgent treatment should be instigated with **ampicillin** 50 mg/kg 6-hourly or **chloramphenicol** 12.5 mg/kg 6-hourly given intravenously if there is any sign of respiratory obstruction.

Dental Significance

Where possible dental treatment should be put off for patients suffering from pharyngitis, and general anaesthetics avoided. Surgeon and dental assistants should wear masks to reduce chance of picking up the infection.

PHTHISIS, see TUBERCULOSIS.

PLEURISY

Inflammation of the pleura may occur with or without underlying lung disease, and has many causes. Pulmonary infection and pulmonary infarction due to embolization are the commonest causes but neoplasia, trauma, and collagen diseases may be responsible. Clinical features are pain on respiration and a pleural rub on auscultation. In addition there may be features of the underlying cause; for example, fever, haemoptysis, or shortness of breath. In general pleurisy is an indication of underlying disease rather than a disease itself, and therefore warrants further investigation. Treatment is that of the underlying cause coupled with prescribing of appropriate analgesics.

Dental Significance

Emergency treatment to ease pain or pre-operative removal of infected teeth is all that will be required in a patient with pleurisy. The question of antibiotic cover should be discussed with the patient's physician. General anaesthetics are best avoided, and if essential administered in hospital.

PLEURODYNIA, see BORNHOLM'S DISEASE.

PLUMMER-VINSON SYNDROME, see ANAEMIA.

PNEUMOCONIOSES (occupational lung disease)

These conditions result from inhalation of inorganic or organic dust in the course of work, leading to a variety of lung disorders, the most common of which are:

ANTHRACOSIS (COAL-WORKERS' PNEUMOCONIOSIS)

This is due to coal dust and usually causes no symptoms except in 1 per cent when extensive fibrosis occurs (progressive massive fibrosis) giving rise to breathlessness and haemoptysis.

SILICOSIS

This results from inhalation of silica-containing dust which causes fibrosis and leads to breathlessness and later haemoptysis.

ASBESTOSIS

This condition results from inhaling asbestos particles and is associated with the serious complication of mesothelioma formation.

Dental Significance

There are no contra-indications to routine dentistry, but general anaesthetics are to be avoided.

PNEUMONIA

This is inflammatory consolidation of the lung and may result from physical or chemical agents. Only infective pneumonias are considered here.

Pneumonias may be classified as primary, occurring in a previously healthy person, or secondary when occurring in association with pre-existing lung disease, influenza, aspiration, or immunological impairment. Symptoms are of fever, cough and often pleuritic pain. Classical lobar pneumonia is seldom seen due to the tendency to prescribe antibiotics early.

Lobar pneumonia in a previously healthy person is usually caused by *Streptococcus pneumoniae* and **penicillin** is the antibiotic of choice. In chronic bronchitics and asthmatics pneumonia is likely to be due to *Pneumococcus* or *Haemophilus influenzae*, when **amoxycillin** should be prescribed. Other primary pneumonias, caused by non-bacterial organisms, viruses, *Mycoplasma, Chlamydia* (psittacosis), *Coxiella burneti* (Q fever), are termed primary atypical pneumonias.

Tetracycline may be effective against several organisms responsible for primary atypical pneumonia.

Dental Significance

It is unlikely that a patient suffering from pneumonia will present for dental treatment.

PNEUMOTHORAX

This is the presence of air in the pleural sac, and may be classified as follows:

spontaneous pneumothorax;
traumatic pneumothorax;
tension pneumothorax.

The majority of pneumothoraces are spontaneous and probably result from rupture of small pulmonary bulli, though often no cause is established. Onset is abrupt with chest pain and shortness of breath. Diagnosis is confirmed with a chest X-ray taken in expiration. Recovery may be spontaneous, but with troublesome symptoms and a large degree of lung collapse a chest drain is advisable to rapidly reflate the lung.

A tension pneumothorax is the most dangerous complication of a pneumothorax. Air accumulates under pressure, collapsing the lung, shifting the mediastinum and causing progressive collapse of the other lung. Without prompt treatment (insertion of a wide-bore needle into the pneumothorax), death ensues.

Traumatic pneumothoraces are seen in association with penetrating chest wounds and may complicate diagnostic or therapeutic needle procedures to the chest.

Pneumothoraces may be recurrent, in which case treatment, either by insertion of irritant material into the pleural cavity or by pleurectomy, is necessary. This is particularly so when pneumothoraces have occurred bilaterally.

Dental Significance

Respiration is hampered and vital capacity reduced, so general anaesthetics should be avoided.

POLIOMYELITIS

This is a virus disease with an incubation period of 7–14 days. There are three types of poliovirus and all gain entry through ingested food or water. Once epidemic in the UK, only sporadic cases in non-immunized persons are now recorded.

The disease starts with fever, headache, and signs of meningeal irritation, which are followed in a number of cases by asymmetrical paralysis of varying degree.

There is no treatment other than strict rest in the initial stages, and symptomatic treatment of the paralysis later.

Life-long immunity is obtained with either IPV (Salk) or OPV (Sabin) vaccine. The latter is more commonly used, 4–5 doses of the oral vaccine being given over the years of childhood and adolescence. Travellers outside Europe, North America, and Australasia are well advised to check that they have been immunized.

Dental Significance

While recent cases are unlikely to be encountered, the dentist may be called to treat patients with varying degrees of paralysis as a result of polio 30 years ago. General dentistry for those in a respirator is quite possible provided adequate suction is available.

POLYARTERITIS NODOSUM

This is a collagen disorder of unknown cause in which focal inflammation of small and medium-sized arteries occurs. It is widespread though occasionally is limited to one organ. In 50 per cent of patients the presenting features are fever, tachycardia, generalized aching, abdominal pain, and weight loss. Presentation may be with specific system involvement, for example asthma, renal failure, neuropathy, coronary artery disease, Raynaud's, and a variety of skin lesions.

The disease may take a fulminating and rapidly fatal course over weeks or months, or may be extremely mild ending in full recovery. Renal and pulmonary involvement carry a poor prognosis. There is no specific treatment, **corticosteroids** being the mainstay of drug treatment together with supportive treatment for complications.

Dental Significance

Oral manifestations seem to be rare though papules in the mouth and oral ulcers have been described. A significant proportion of patients suffering from this condition are hepatitis B antigen-positive and routine dental treatment should be undertaken with this in mind. (see LIVER DISEASE, HEPATITIS).

General anaesthetics should be avoided.

POLYCYTHAEMIA, see MYELOPROLIFERATIVE DISORDERS.

POLYMYALGIA RHEUMATICA

This is a muscular rheumatism seen in old people and characterized by pain; stiffness in the neck, shoulders, and back; and occasionally low-grade fever. The striking laboratory finding is a greatly raised ESR. It is frequently associated with cranial arteritis. Systemic steroids result in a dramatic response.

Dental Significance

Jaw-ache, with tenderness of the masseter and temporal muscles, is a common symptom. Dentists should enquire whether corticosteroids have been taken during the last 12 months and act accordingly (see ADRENAL INSUFFICIENCY).

POLYMYOSITIS, see DERMATOMYOSITIS.

POLYNEUROPATHY

Simultaneous impairment of multiple peripheral nerves most commonly results in a distal and symmetrical lower motor neurone weakness with disturbance of sensation in some areas. There are many causes:

- Infection
  - Diphtheria
  - Leprosy
  - Viral
- Metabolic
  - Diabetes
  - Uraemia
  - Alcohol
  - Amyloid
- Poisons
  - Heavy metals
  - Organic poisons
- Vascular and collagen diseases
- Carcinomata

It is essential to try and establish the underlying cause of the neuropathy, for although with some causes—such as carcinoma and collagen diseases—the changes are likely to be irreversible, in others—such as alcohol, heavy metals, and viral—full recovery may occur.

Dental Significance

Routine dentistry must be tailored to that which the patient can tolerate.

General anaesthetics are inadvisable.

Dentists should appreciate their susceptibility to chronic mercury poisoning and be aware of the clinical picture it produces. The neurological symptoms include tremor of the arms and legs with deterioration of the handwriting, as well as psychic disturbances which are characterized by loss of decision, self-consciousness, timidity, and depression. In addition there may be frequent headaches, gingivitis, and gastrointestinal symptoms.

Diagnosis is made by analysis of blood and urine levels of mercury.

THE PORPHYRIAS

This is a group of conditions resulting from abnormal porphyrin metabolism. The major groups are erythropoietic and hepatic, based on the anatomical source of the products of porphyrin metabolism.

ERYTHROPOIETIC PORPHYRIAS

The rare congenital form gives rise to severe photosensitivity, vesicle formation, with subsequent scarring. Deformity of the fingers, hypertrichosis, a pinkish discoloration of the teeth, haemolytic anaemia, and splenomegaly are seen.

Erythropoietic protoporphyrin is commoner and causes intense pruritis and burning of the skin, urticaria, and weal formation.

HEPATIC PORPHYRIAS

Some of these are due to a genetic abnormality but in many there is no evidence of this and various toxins are responsible. They may present in one or two ways: either with alimentary, cardiovascular, and nervous system symptoms or with symptoms confined to photosensitivity and skin lesions. In acute intermittent porphyria, which is genetically determined, skin manifestations do not occur and symptoms are abdominal pain, motor weakness and paralysis, sensory disturbance, occasionally epilepsy, and tachycardia. In porphyria cutanea tarda cutaneous symptoms predominate with lesions in light-exposed areas, increased pigmentation of skin and hair, and vesicle formation, with secondary infection leading to scarring. The skin is very fragile, minor trauma leading to vesicle formation. Hepatomegaly and jaundice may be seen in some patients, and are often associated with high alcohol intake.

Treatment is preventative, care being taken to avoid precipitating factors. During an attack symptomatic treatment is necessary.

Dental Significance

In erythropoietic porphyria the deciduous and permanent teeth have a brown–pink discoloration (erythrodontia) which is fluorescent under UV light. Periodontal disease is common and the presence of anaemia must be considered if a general anaesthetic is planned.

Hepatic porphyrias carry no oral manifestations, but **barbiturates** are frequently precipitators of intermittent porphyria and should be avoided.

PREGNANCY

Dental Significance

Pregnancy gingivitis, which is the main oral manifestation, is thought to result from increased capillary permeability by reason of raised progesterone levels in the blood. It may become evident as early as the second month of pregnancy but quickly diminishes after parturition. Efficient plaque control is important and remains the only treatment.

X-ray examinations during pregnancy should be avoided. Foetal damage is more likely during the early stages of development and all women of child-bearing age should be questioned about the probability of their being pregnant and X-rays postponed if menstruation is overdue.

A year never passes without another drug coming under suspicion of causing foetal abnormalities. To date none used in dentistry has been implicated, but it is a wise precaution to stick to well-tried methods of pain and infection control during this time.

General anaesthetics can be administered to pregnant patients with a few precautions. The third month of pregnancy is best avoided, especially in those with a history of miscarriage, and also the last few weeks when a large gravid uterus can cause respiratory and circulatory embarrassment. A simple blood pressure reading should be taken at the previous appointment and patients in excess of 150/90 referred for a medical opinion prior to administration. Opiates should not be used as premedication, and the anaesthetic should be conducted without any obstruction to the airway, using anaesthetic gases containing 50 per cent oxygen.

During the terminal weeks of pregnancy partial obstruction of the inferior vena cava from pressure by the uterus can be provoked with the patient in the supine position. Dentists who work on supine patients should appreciate this and allow these patients to sit up from time to time during sessions of conservative or operative dentistry.

PROGRESSIVE MUSCULAR ATROPHY, see MUSCULAR DYSTROPHIES.

PSEUDOMEMBRANOUS COLITIS, see COLITIS.

PSITTACOSIS

This is a specific infection of birds caused by an obligate intracellular bacterium *Chlamydia psittaci*. This can be transmitted to man to give an asymptomatic infection, a mild 'flu-like disease, or a serious pneumonic illness with high fever, headache, cough, myalgia, and significant mortality.

Tetracycline is the treatment of choice.

Dental Significance

None.

PSORIASIS

The cause of this common skin condition is unknown, but it is frequently precipitated by stress or infection and is more common in the winter months. The typical red patches covered with silvery scales can occur anywhere on the body but are more frequent on the knees and elbows. A pustular eruption is also described.

Treatment is with local application of **hydrocortisone** ointment 1 per cent, **coal tar** in a paste or paint, and **dithranol.** PUVA (psoralen and ultraviolet light) is used when the condition is widespread.

Dental Significance

Small white lesions on the gingivae, and geographic tongue, have been described in patients with psoriasis.

PSYCHIATRIC DISORDERS

It is not within the scope of this book to describe psychiatric disease and its treatment. The degree of co-operation for dentistry can only be assessed by enquiries of relatives, doctors, and nurses, who are usually helpful in suggesting a line of approach. In the end it falls to the dentist to decide what treatment is advisable and how best it can be carried out. The majority of psychiatric patients present few difficulties, but for a small number dental treatment is only possible after heavy sedation or under anaesthesia.

Almost all patients with psychiatric disorders will be receiving medical treatment and it is important for the dentist to find out the name and dosage of the drugs they are being given. Tricyclic anti-depressants, such as **amitriptyline** (*Lentizol*$_{GB}$,

Tryptizol$_{GB}$, *Amitil*$_{US}$), and **imipramine** (*Tofranil*$_{GB,US}$) prevent the uptake of catecholamines and potentiate the action of **adrenaline** and **nor-adrenaline**. Hence it is wise to avoid using a local anaesthetic with these. Monoamine-oxidase inhibitors, such as **phenelzine** (*Nardil*$_{GB,US}$) and **iproniazid** (*Marsilid*$_{GB}$) are said to be free of interaction with catecholamines but interact with other sypathomimetic non-catecholamine drugs. However it is safer to adopt the same routine with local anaesthesia and be careful not to prescribe any preparation containing **amphetamine, ephedrine**, or a narcotic analgesic, if the patient has been on these drugs within the last 14 days. **Phenytoin** (*Epanutin*$_{GB}$, *Dilantin*$_{US}$) is sometimes given for psychiatric disorders. Its effect on the gums is a problem (see EPILEPSY) and it is known to potentiate the action of **diazepam** (*Valium*$_{GB,US}$).

PULMONARY EMBOLISM, see EMBOLISM.

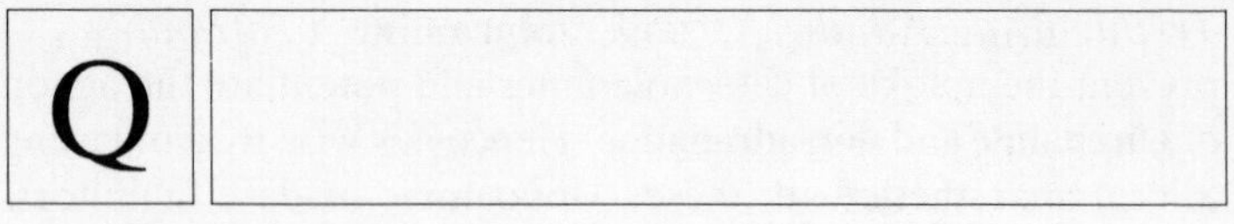

QUINSY, see **TONSILLITIS**.

R

RAMSAY-HUNT SYNDROME, see BELL'S PALSY.

Q R

RAYNAUD'S PHENOMENON

The features of Raynaud's phenomenon are intermittent pallor and cyanosis of the extremities brought on by cold with return to normal colour between attacks. These changes result from an excessive vasoconstrictor response to the cold. Raynaud's may occur as an isolated phenomenon usually with no long-term sequelae. However, it complicates conditions such as scleroderma, systemic lupus erythematosus, and polyarteritis nodosum when the prognosis is less favourable and related to that of the associated disease.

Treatment includes protection from the cold and wet, the use of alpha-adrenergic blocking agents such as **phenoxy benzamine** (*Dibenyline*$_{GB}$, *Dibenzyline*$_{US}$) and, when medical management fails, cervical sympathectomy.

Dental Significance

Delayed healing of extraction sockets has been reported.

REITER'S SYNDROME

This condition which causes inflammation of the urethra, conjunctivae and joints, occurs predominantly in males, most commonly between the ages of 20 and 30. The three parts of the body become involved in the order mentioned, with a 3- or 4-day interval before spreading to the next. The causative agent is unknown. There is no effective treatment, but the condition usually resolves on its own.

Dental Significance

Oral lesions in the form of small elevated red spots or vesicles occur in approximately 25 per cent of cases. They are seen on the gums and buccal mucosa and are usually painless. Involvement of the temporomandibular joint with the arthritis is rare.

RENAL DISEASE

GLOMERULO-NEPHRITIS

The clinical presentation of glomerular disease is extremely variable, the main features being proteinuria, haematuria, and hypertension. The following syndromes are recognized modes of presentation:

acute nephritis;
nephrotic syndrome;
asymptomatic proteinuria;
recurrent haematuria;
hypertension;
acute and chronic renal failure.

Definitive diagnosis depends on renal biopsy. Glomerulonephritis may be primary or secondary to underlying disease, such as systemic lupus erythematosus, diabetes, and amyloid. The commoner and clinically more important types are:

MEMBRANOUS GLOMERULONEPHRITIS

Diffuse uniform thickening of the glomerular capillary wall is the histological feature of this type of glomerulonephritis. It usually presents as the nephrotic syndrome the features of which are hypoalbuminaemia, gross proteinuria, hypercholesterolaemia, and oedema. It may complicate certain infections—malaria, hepatitis B, and syphilis—and may result from certain drugs, penicillamine, and gold. Other conditions, such as Hodgkin's disease, carcinoma of breast, sarcoid, and diabetes mellitus may also give rise to membranous glomerulonephritis, but frequently no cause is established.

Management includes a high-protein, low-sodium diet, diuretic therapy, and regular follow-up.

MINIMAL LESION GLOMERULONEPHRITIS

This syndrome is characterized by severe proteinuria and only minimal abnormality on renal biopsy. It occurs in children and its cause is not known. It runs a relapsing course and carries a good prognosis, spontaneous remission occurring in 30 per cent. Treatment includes diuretic therapy and systemic steroids.

DIFFUSE PROLIFERATIVE GLOMERULONEPHRITIS

The hallmark of this condition is an increase in the number of cells in the glomerular tuft. Presentation is extremely variable but usually takes the form of an acute nephritis or occasionally nephrotic syndrome. It may occur at any age with no sex preponderance. The majority of cases are thought to be due to deposition of small, soluble, circulating immune complexes in glomerular capillary walls as seen in post-streptococcal glomerulonephritis.

POST-STREPTOCOCCAL GLOMERULONEPHRITIS

This type of proliferative glomerulonephritis develops as a result of immune complex formation following streptococcal infection, usually in children of school age.

Clinical features are frequently those of an acute nephritis with oliguria, haematuria, hypertension, and impaired renal function. Full recovery occurs in 80–90 per cent but a few have persisting minor renal abnormalities and death occasionally occurs in the acute phase. Management involves treatment of the acute infection, control of hypertension, close observation of renal function, and long-term follow-up.

FOCAL GLOMERULONEPHRITIS

As its name implies, this is a patchy disease of the glomeruli, frequently associated with systemic diseases such as systemic lupus erythematosus, Henoch-Schönlein purpura, and sub-acute bacterial endocarditis. It presents with haematuria and sometimes acute nephritis or nephrotic syndrome. Clinical features are extremely variable. The cause is not known but the prognosis is usually good.

PYELONEPHRITIS

Chronic pyelonephritis is a common cause of renal failure, occurring more often in women than men. It may occur as a primary event or secondary to functional or anatomical renal abnormalities. Intestinal bacteria, *Escherichia coli, Proteus vulgaris,* and *Pseudomonas,* are the commonest causes of infection. The condition may be asymptomatic or give rise to frequency and dysuria. In an acute attack malaise, fever, rigors, vomiting, and headache dominate the picture, together with marked renal tenderness on examination. Preventative treatment is important as there is no cure for established chronic pyelonephritis. Personal hygiene, prompt treatment of infection, and exclusion of anatomical abnormalities when recurrent urinary infections occur, are all important.

ACUTE RENAL FAILURE

Pre-renal, renal, and post-renal factors can lead to acute renal failure. Hypovolaemia from saline depletion, haemorrhage, or burns are the major pre-renal cause and, with prompt treatment, the prognosis is good. Renal causes include nephrotoxins, renal ischaemia, septicaemia, acute glomerulonephritis, and arterial and venous thromboses. Obstructions to urine outflow from whatever cause will lead ultimately to post-renal failure. The clinical features of renal failure result from electrolyte and fluid disturbances, and are anorexia, nausea, vomiting, dyspnoea, circulatory overload, drowsiness, confusion, occasionally convulsions, and coma. Secondary infection is a major hazard.

Treatment depends on the cause. Once renal failure is established management should be in an intensive care unit, special attention being given to fluid balance, electrolyte intake, acid–base balance, nutrition, and prevention of infection. Dialysis will be necessary when there is a high blood urea, high blood potassium, fluid overload, or severe metabolic acidosis.

CHRONIC RENAL FAILURE

The major causes of chronic renal failure in Europe are glomerulonephritis (48 per cent), pyelonephritis (20 per cent), and cystic disease of the kidney (8 per cent). Symptoms are multiple and varied and include fatigue, dyspnoea, anorexia, nausea, vomiting, diarrhoea, bleeding, and occasionally fits.

Once diagnosed, careful consideration must be given to the control of hypertension, intercurrent illness, gastrointestinal upsets, and avoiding nephrotoxic drugs.

Suitability of patients for eventual haemodialysis or transplantation should be considered early on. Management consists initially of control by dietary measures. Ultimately dialysis will be necessary; indications include fluid overload, hyperkalaemia, pericarditis, neurological complications, and increasing malaise.

Dental Significance

Disease of the kidneys produces no signs in the mouth until renal failure sets in. With acute renal failure a dry brown-furred tongue is to be found, accompanied by gingival haemorrhages, while in the chronic condition exudative stomatitis, oral ulcers, and keratosis may be seen. The oral features improve with successful treatment of the general condition, but in the meantime advice and assistance with oral hygiene is important, together with local treatment of *Candida* or bacterial mouth infection.

Some drugs are nephrotoxic and should not be used in patients with renal disease. They include **tetracyclines, talampicillin** (*Talpen*$_{GB}$), and **cephaloridine** (*Ceporex*$_{GB}$, *Loridine*$_{US}$), while the action of others, such as hypnotics, sedatives, and tranquillizers, may be extended so they should be prescribed with caution.

Penicillin, ampicillin, and **erythromycin** are safe but **metronidazole** (*Flagyl*$_{GB,US}$) should be prescribed in reduced dosage. **Aspirin** and **diflunisal** (*Dolobid*$_{GB}$) are best avoided, but **paracetamol** is safe to use. Concurrent or previous treatment with steroids demands special precautions (see ADRENAL INSUFFICIENCY.

RHEUMATIC FEVER

This inflammatory disease results from pharyngeal infection with a group A Streptococcus. It occurs most commonly between the ages of 5 and 15 years in approximately 3 per cent of those with exudative streptococcal pharyngitis. Those who have had rheumatic fever are more likely to have further attacks than the general population. The disease is multi-system, affecting heart, joints, central nervous system, skin, and subcutaneous tissue. Clinical manifestations are fever, migratory polyarthritis, and carditis but Sydenham's chorea, subcutaneous nodules, and erythema marginatum are common features. Although joint symptoms may dominate the clinical picture, the serious sequelae relate to valvular and myocardial heart damage, death occasionally occurring in the acute phase.

Treatment in the acute phase is with intramuscular **procaine penicillin** (600,000 units daily), given to eliminate the streptococcus while symptomatic treatment is given for arthralgia. Preventative treatment is important, especially in those with a history of rheumatic fever who should have long-term prophylactic **penicillin** (200,000 units twice daily) or **sulphadiazine** (1 g daily). All patients under 18 years should receive such treatment. Over 18 years the duration of treatment is debatable but 5 years is recommended. Prevention of the initial rheumatic attack depends on prompt vigorous treatment of group A streptococcal infections.

Dental Significance

Antibiotic cover is required for any dental procedure likely to cause a bacteraemia in patients who may be suffering from rheumatic fever or whose heart valves may have been damaged by the disease in the past (see HEART DISEASE, infective,

SUBACUTE BACTERIAL ENDOCARDITIS). General anaesthetics should not be given without an assessment by a physician.

RHEUMATOID ARTHRITIS

The cause of this chronic systemic disease is unknown. Its main feature is a symmetrical inflammatory arthritis which may be accompanied by haematological, pulmonary, neurological, and cardiovascular manifestations. The peak age of onset is in the fourth decade and a genetic predisposition is suggested by the association with the histocompatibility antigen HLA DW4. Onset is usually insidious; fatigue, weakness, stiffness, and myalgia preceding the development of joint swelling. The proximal interphalangeal, metacarpophalangeal, wrist, knee, elbow, and ankle joints are most commonly involved. Atlanto-axial joint involvement may result in instability of the upper cervical spine. Temporomandibular joint involvement may interfere with mastication and pain may be referred to the middle ear and throat.

A diffuse interstitial fibrosis may affect the lungs. Heart disease is uncommon but amyloid may complicate the condition, leading to renal failure.

Ten to twenty per cent of patients have a complete remission or mild intermittent disease while 10 per cent progress inexorably to crippling arthritis. Careful continuous medical supervision is essential, aiming to maintain the patient's ability to function as normally as possible. The objects of treatment are to reduce inflammation and pain, maintain motion and strength, and prevent joint deformity by appropriate physiotherapy, anti-inflammatory drugs, splints, physical rest, and orthopaedic surgery.

Dental Significance

The temporomandibular joint is affected in over 50 per cent of patients suffering from this disease. Apart from general treatment, sufferers may be helped by the fitting of a soft bite-raising appliance carefully constructed to keep the posterior teeth apart by about 3 mm.

Sjögren's syndrome of xerostomia and conjunctivitis sicca, with or without enlargement of the salivary and lacrymal glands, sometimes accompanies the condition.

Recent treatment with steroids must be taken into account when extractions or anaesthetics are being planned (see ADRENAL INSUFFICIENCY).

RICKETS, see VITAMIN DEFICIENCIES.

RINGWORM, see TINEA.

RUBELLA (German Measles)

Rubella is a mild infectious fever with an incubation period of 2–3 weeks. Its characteristics are a rash of pink macules which remain discrete, and enlargement of the occipital lymph nodes.

The danger of rubella lies in the high incidence of foetal abnormality if it is contracted during the first 4 months of pregnancy. For those who have not had rubella in childhood immunity can be obtained from vaccination with a single dose of attenuated rubella virus. It must not be given if already pregnant.

Dental Significance

By reason of frequent close contact with children there is an occupational hazard of rubella in dentistry. All non-immune female dentists and surgery staff should be vaccinated. In the event of pregnant non-immune personnel coming in contact with the disease, high-titre immunoglobulin should be given as soon as possible.

S

SALIVARY CALCULI

Salivary calculi are three times more common in the submandibular gland and its duct than in the other salivary glands. They cause pain on eating and their presence is frequently complicated by infection of the gland. Near the orifice of the duct they can be localized by palpation, while more distally an X-ray (angled to avoid superimposition of the mandible) will be required to disclose their presence. Stones in the duct can usually be removed by intra-oral surgery but if situated in the substance of the gland the submandibular gland must be removed via an external approach.

Dental Significance

Small stones impacted near the duct orifice can be removed by the dentist quite simply with a small infiltration of local anaesthetic. After clamping the duct distally to stop them slipping back the duct is incised over them and they are eased out.

SARCOIDOSIS

This is a multi-system granulomatous disorder of unknown aetiology commonly affecting young adults and presenting most frequently with bilateral hilar lymphadenopathy, pulmonary infiltration, and skin and eye lesions. Other organs commonly involved are peripheral lymph nodes, liver, spleen, parotids, muscle, heart, mucous membrane, and nervous system.

The clinical picture is very variable.

Diagnosis may be incidental on a routine chest X-ray or the disease may present with severe incapacitating symptoms, including fever, weight loss, fatigue, and general malaise. Dyspnoea accompanies pulmonary involvement, uveitis and keratoconjunctivitis sicca are features of eye involvement. Skin lesions occur in 30 per cent of patients and include erythema nodosum, erythematous raised infiltrated lesions, or non-specific papules or plaques. Variable neurological lesions include isolated facial weakness, peripheral neuropathy, and disordered swallowing.

Diagnosis is made on the clinical features and may be supported by histology and a positive Kveim reaction. No treatment may be necessary but steroids are the treatment of choice with progressive pulmonary disease, active ocular disease, central nervous system involvement, hypercalcaemia, myocardial disease, and persistent systemic illness. In general the prognosis for sarcoid is good, 80–85 per cent recovering from the disease. Occasionally patients die from cardiac or renal involvement but in the majority the outcome depends on pulmonary involvement where, in a small percentage, pulmonary fibrosis is progressive and disabling.

Dental Significance

Dark red sarcoid nodules are sometimes found on the palate or elsewhere in the mouth. They are painless and seldom ulcerate. As with other diseases treated with steroids, special precautions must be taken when extractions or general anaesthetics are planned (see ADRENAL INSUFFICIENCY). If pulmonary fibrosis has developed general anaesthetics should be conducted in hospital.

SCABIES

The disease is caused by infection with a mite (*Sarcoptes*), picked up by close body contact or through infected clothes or bedding. The short burrows of the female mite can be found in the epidermis of the limbs and trunk but seldom on the head and neck. Itching is intense and hence secondary infection is common as a result of scratching.

Treatment consists of thorough overall cleaning, followed by two applications of **benzyl benzoate** (*Ascabiol*$_{GB}$) or **gamma benzene hydrochloride** (*Quellada*$_{GB}$). Residual irritation may continue for several days. Clothing and bedding should be thoroughly washed or dry-cleaned.

Dental Significance

The burrows being uncommon on the head and neck, it is most unlikely that a dentist will pick up scabies from an infected patient.

SCARLET FEVER

This disorder reults from streptococcal production of erythrogenic toxin. The infection is usually pharyngeal and the rash develops within 2 days, spreading to involve the whole body, sparing the palms and soles. Punctate erythema and petechiae occur on the soft palate. The tongue is coated initially but this is shed to leave the typical raw 'red raspberry tongue'. The rash lasts 4–5 days and is followed by extensive desquamation.

Dental Significance

None.

SCLERODERMA, see SYSTEMIC SCLEROSIS.

SCURVY, see VITAMIN DEFICIENCIES.

SHINGLES, see HERPES ZOSTER.

SICKLE CELL ANAEMIA, see ANAEMIA.

SILICOSIS, see PNEUMOCONIOSIS.

SINUSITIS

Infection of the maxillary and frontal sinuses usually follows a cold. Initially the agent is a virus but secondary bacterial infection follows. Pain is felt over the sinus involved, and with infection of the frontal sinus there may be swelling above the eye.

Treatment is with inhalations of **tinct. benz. co.** (friar's balsam) 5 ml in 500 ml of hot water and decongestant nose drops run in to reach the ostium of the sinus involved. Examples of these are **ephedrine** nose drops, **oxymetazoline** (*Alfrazine*$_{\text{GB}}$, *Iliadinene*$_{\text{GB}}$, *Alfrin*$_{\text{US}}$), and **xylometazoline** (*Otrivine*$_{\text{GB}}$, *Otrivin*$_{\text{US}}$), but they should not be prescribed for patients on treatment with monoamine-oxidase inhibitors or antihypertensive agents. Antibiotics are required for frontal sinusitis and maxillary sinusitis which does not respond to these measures.

Chronic sinusitis requires operative treatment.

Dental Significance

Because of the proximity of the maxillary sinus to the apices of the upper premolar and molar teeth, patients with sinusitis may visit the dentist, complaining of toothache. The recent history of a cold with persistent nasal congestion should alert the dentist to the possible cause of their discomfort.

SJÖGREN'S SYNDROME

The condition occurs predominantly in females of middle age and is caused by lymphocyte infiltration of the lacrymal and salivary glands greatly reducing their natural secretions. It is frequently associated with rheumatoid arthritis and other connective tissue diseases. Patients complain of prickly inflamed eyes, dysphagia, and a dry mouth, and on examination the tongue is found dry, shiny, and fissured and there may be oral ulceration and candida infection.

Local treatment consists of keeping the eyes and mouth lubricated with drops and mouthwashes containing 1 or 2 per cent **methylcellulose**, **glycerine** lozenges, and lemon sweets to encourage saliva flow. Immunosuppressive agents and corticosteroids may help but are usually reserved for severe cases. Malignant lymphoma is a complication.

Dental Significance

In those with teeth an increase in caries is an inevitable sequel, and advice and assistance with oral hygiene is important. The edentulous will experience difficulty in keeping dentures in place.

STEVENS–JOHNSON SYNDROME

This is a severe form of erythema multiformae with development of extensive exudative, bullous, and erosive cutaneous lesions involving the mouth, conjunctivae, cornea, and genitals. Pannus formation and blindness may result. The condition is extremely distressing and urgent treatment with systemic steroids is required to prevent serious ocular complications.

Dental Significance

The lesions may occur anywhere in the mouth but are seen with greatest regularity on the lips. They start as vesicles which rapidly coalesce and break down to large painful ulcers whose base is covered by a slough or pseudomembrane. On the lips haemorrhagic crusting will be seen. Treatment is with **hydrocortisone** in the form of 1 per cent ointment on the lips and as 2.5 mg lozenges (*Corlan*$_{GB}$) or **triamcinolone** paste (*Adcortyl*$_{GB}$, *Kenalog*$_{US}$) in orobase in the mouth. **Chlorhexidine** 0.2 per cent mouthwash (*Corsodyl*$_{GB}$) will help to prevent secondary infection.

STOKES–ADAMS ATTACKS, see **HEART DISEASE (Dysrhythmia).**

STROKE, see **VASCULAR DISEASE.**

SUBACUTE BACTERIAL ENDOCARDITIS, see **HEART DISEASE (Infective), SUBACUTE BACTERIAL ENDOCARDITIS.**

SUBACUTE COMBINED DEGENERATION OF THE CORD

This is the most serious consequence of deficiency of vitamin B12 and occurs in association with pernicious anaemia. The white matter of the spinal cord degenerates leading to progressive irreversible damage to the posterior and lateral columns and there is an associated peripheral neuropathy.

First symptoms are usually numbness or tingling of the feet, leading to unsteadiness on walking and progressive weakness. Examination reveals weakness, loss of vibration and position sense, absent knee and ankle reflexes, and extensor plantar responses. Romberg's sign is positive. Untreated the condition progresses to paralysis. Optic atrophy and mental changes are a feature in a few people. It is essential to be aware of this complication of B12 deficiency and to treat promptly with intramuscular injections of **hydroxocobalamin** (1000 mg on alternate days for a month then monthly permanently) before irreversible neurological damage occurs.

Dental Significance

The manifestations of the condition should be borne in mind when a patient presents with glossitis and recurrent oral ulceration. These painful symptoms may lead a patient to take advice while neglecting the early neurological features of the disease.

SUB-ARACHNOID HAEMORRHAGE, see INTRACRANIAL HAEMORRHAGE.

SYDENHAM'S CHOREA, see CHOREA.

SYNCOPE

This is a brief, transient, and totally reversible loss of consciousness due to acute arterial hypotension. The most common form is vasovagal syncope (fainting) when the patient is usually in the upright position; feels 'faint'; and becomes pale, sweaty, and tachpnoeic. The syncope is accompanied by a bradycardia and hypotension. Recovery is rapid in the recumbent position.

Dental Significance

There must be few dentists who have not experienced vasovagal syncope in a patient before or after a local anaesthetic injection. The immediate treatment is to lay the patient flat and recovery is rapid. The danger of the condition is when it is unnoticed and the patient restrained in the upright position with resulting cerebral anoxia. There is strong evidence to show that several deaths have occurred under anaesthesia in an upright dental chair from this cause. The authors believe that general dental anaesthetics should only be given to patients in the supine position and that those who have just had a local anaesthetic injection should not be left unattended.

SYPHILIS

Syphilis is now less common than other venereal diseases but remains an important medical problem. It results from infection by the spirochaete *Treponema pallidum*. Incubation ranges from 9 to 90 days. The primary lesion develops from a macule to a papule and eventually to an ulcer (chancre) which is painless and usually on the genitals but occasionally extra-genital, on the lips, tongue, fingers, nipples, or anus. Secondary syphilis develops within 6–8 weeks of the primary sore and is a generalized non-irritant dull red rash. There may follow a symptomless stage (latent syphilis) prior to development of late or tertiary syphilis. Late syphilis may occur within 5 years of the primary sore or may appear much later, when involvement of the skin, cardiovascular system, central nervous system, or skeleton may occur. The late lesion or gumma may affect the skin, various viscera, and mucous membranes. The tibia is the commonest bone involved. Aortitis may lead to aortic aneurysm formation and aortic incompetence. Neurosyphilis may give rise to meningovascular involvement with headaches, cranial nerve involvement, and cerebrovascular accidents due to arterial involvement. Spinal column involvement causes tabes dorsalis with impaired proprioception, and vibration sense, muscular hypotonia, Argyll–Robertson pupils, ataxia, lightning pains in the legs, and transient severe abdominal pain. Generalized cortical involvement leads to general paralysis of the insane (GPI). Diagnosis is made clinically and confirmed in the early stages by demonstrating the spirochaete, and in all stages by serological tests (VDRL, FTA, and TPI).

The patient with late syphilis is no longer infectious.

Penicillin is the mainstay of treatment (daily intramuscular **procaine penicillin** 1–2 mega-units for 10 days in the early stages of acquired infection). For late syphilis 20 mega-units are given in 3 weeks. Results in neurosyphilis are variable, good in meningovascular disease, unpredictable in GPI, and poor in tabes dorsalis.

Dental Significance

Though tertiary syphilis is less common the dentist may still meet the condition in the primary or secondary stage.

A primary chancre on the lips or tongue presents as a round or oval ulcer 1–2 cm across with a red indurated base. Unless secondarily infected it causes little pain, but is always accompanied by enlargement of the regional lymph nodes. In secondary syphilis raised grey–white patches are to be seen on the fauces, tongue, and palate, which break down and coalesce to form the snail-track ulcer. The lymph nodes are enlarged. Both the stages are infections to the dentist and subsequent patients. If suspicious, avoid examining the lesions with unprotected hands and make sure all instruments and utensils are effectively sterilized.

In tertiary syphilis gummas are sometimes found on the palate and tongue and are distinguished by their characteristic punched-out appearance. Chronic glossitis and leukoplakia are other oral manifestations of this stage.

SYRINGOMYELIA

This uncommon condition results from cavitation in the brain stem and spinal cord, possibly relating to a congenital abnormality. Dissociated sensory loss with preserved sensation to touch but loss of pain and temperature sensation is characteristic. Muscular atrophy occurs predominantly in the upper limbs. Surgery can halt progression so early diagnosis is important.

Dental Significance

There may be loss of pain and thermal sensation over the distribution of the trigeminal nerve with weakness of the palate and tongue if the cavitation extends into the brain stem.

SYSTEMIC LUPUS ERYTHEMATOSUS, see LUPUS ERYTHEMATOSUS.

SYSTEMIC SCLEROSIS

Progressive systemic sclerosis is a disorder of connective tissue leading to fibrosis of the skin (scleroderma) and various internal organs, notably the gastrointestinal tract, lungs, heart, and kidneys. Its cause is unknown.

The onset is insidious, often with Raynaud's phenomenon, then symmetrical swelling and stiffening of the fingers. The skin changes to become tight, firm, and bound to underlying subcutaneous tissue.

The hands, arms, face, and upper trunk are mainly involved. The facial features appear pinched and the mouth tight and narrowed. Gastrointestinal involvement leads to reflux oesophagitis, dysphagia, and malabsorption. Cough and dyspnoea herald pulmonary involvement. Cardiac dysrhythmias and various degrees of heart block indicate cardiac involvement. Renal failure is the main cause of death.

Diagnosis is clinical. There is no specific treatment and most patients pursue a progressive downhill course.

Dental Significance

Reduced facial movement and a mask-like expression result from fibrosis in the skin of the face. The lips lose mobility, being either drawn back from the anterior teeth or 'pursed' due to circumoral constriction. The tongue loses mobility and patients suffer from difficulty in feeding and swallowing. There is an increase in caries and periodontal disease. Limited mouth opening adds difficulties to routine dentistry, and dryness of the mouth and fibrosis may cause problems with the wearing of dentures. Advice and assistance with oral hygiene is of great importance.

General anaesthetics are to be avoided.

T

TEMPORAL ARTERITIS, see CRANIAL ARTERITIS.

TETANUS

The causative organism is *Clostridium tetani*, the spores of which are to be found in soil, dust, clothing, and the intestinal tract of animals and man. They enter the body with penetrating wounds. Because of the strict anaerobic conditions needed for growth, tetanus is fortunately rare despite the ubiquity of the organism.

After an incubation period varying from a few days to 2–3 weeks the commonest early symptoms are trismus and pain with stiffness in the neck, back, and abdomen. In moderate and severe cases generalized muscle spasm with opisthotonus and cyanosis develop within 24 hours.

Special tetanus units are equipped for treatment, which includes large doses of antitoxin, antibiotics to prevent pulmonary infection, and scoline and general anaesthesia to control the spasms. The survival rate is only 50 per cent.

Prophylaxis should be given to all infants in the form of triple vaccine during their first year with one or two boosters in later childhood. For an immunized person a further dose of toxoid should be given following a susceptible injury, while a person not immunized will require 250–500 units of human antitetanus immunoglobulin.

Dental Significance

Soil- and dirt-contaminated wounds of the face and mouth may be an entry portal for the organism, and it is the duty of dentists to check the immunity of a patient and act accordingly.

TETANY

This is a syndrome manifested by flexor spasm at the wrist and ankle (carpopedal spasm), muscle twitching, and cramps resulting from low serum calcium or metabolic or respiratory alkalosis.

Dental Significance

None.

T

THALASSAEMIA, see ANAEMIA.

THROMBOCYTHAEMIA, see MYELOPROLIFERATIVE DISORDERS.

THROMBOCYTOPENIA

There are many causes of a low platelet count. Spontaneous bleeding is uncommon if the platelet count is the only abnormality unless the count falls to very low levels, 20,000/mm^3 or less. A relatively low platelet count is, however, of significance when surgical procedures are envisaged.

Low counts result from either failure of platelet production, for example marrow aplasia and neoplastic involvement of the may occur due to drug sensitivity, disseminated intravascular coagulation, systemic lupus erythematosus, massive blood transfusion, and hypersplenism.

Dental Significance

Small submucosal haemorrhages are frequently found on the palate and there may be bleeding from the gingivae.

There should be consultation with a view to platelet transfusion before extractions are undertaken.

THRUSH, see CANDIDA INFECTION.

THYROID DISEASE

HYPERTHYROIDISM

The two common causes of hyperthyroidism are: primary, where the gland is diffusely enlarged due to excessive stimulation by abnormal circulatory immunoglobulins; and secondary, due to excess production of thyroid hormone by hyperactive thyroid nodules.

In young people the classical features of weight loss, hyperactivity, tremor, heat intolerance, and sweating are too well known to need elaborating. In the elderly, cardiac dysrhythmias and failure may be the sole features, and diagnosis may be missed. Diagnosis is clinical, confirmed by a high serum T4 together with a T3 uptake test which allows derivation of the free T4 index, the most helpful single result.

The forms of treatment vary.

Antithyroid drugs: **Carbimazole** (*Neo-mercazole*$_{\text{GB}}$) or **methimazole** (*Tapazole*$_{\text{US}}$) is most commonly used commencing with 30 mg/day reducing to a maintenance dose of 5–15 mg/day and continuing for 12–18 months. Immediate control of symptoms alone can be achieved by the use of beta-adrenergic blockers such as **propranolol** (*Inderal*$_{GB,US}$). When drug treatment fails in the under-45s (child-bearing age), partial thyroidectomy is the treatment of choice. Over 45 years with failed drug treatment, radio-iodine (^{131}I) is given for permanent suppression of the gland.

Dental Significance

There are no oral manifestations of hyperthyroidism and no contra-indications to routine dentistry, but general anaesthetics should be avoided and, if essential, administered in hospital.

HYPOTHYROIDISM

This may result from primary failure of the gland or be secondary to hypothalamic or pituitary disease. Primary failure may be due to idiopathic atrophy, deficient thyroid hormone synthesis, autoimmune disease (Hashimoto's), thyroiditis, surgical removal, malignant infiltration, or irradiation (^{131}I). Though very familiar, the clinical features are often overlooked. The gross features, gruff voice, slowness of movement and expression, and puffy sallow features are obvious. Other, frequently missed, features include anaemia, mental changes and psychoses, alopecia, dry skin, menorrhagia, ataxia, polyneuritis, and carpal tunnel syndrome. Diagnosis is confirmed by a low serum T4 and high TSH levels in primary hypothyroidism. **L-thyroxine sodium** (*Eltroxin*$_{GB}$, *Choloxin*$_{GB,US}$, *Synthroid*$_{US}$) is given (100–200 mg/day) taking particular care in the elderly who may develop cardiac complications and thus should be started on a smaller dose (50 mg/day) initially.

Certain special problems arise in hypothyroidism. Myxoedema coma is rare but often fatal. Neonatal hypothyroidism must be diagnosed early to prevent mental damage.

Dental Significance

In long-standing hypothyroidism swelling of the tongue is common, and in the young this is accompanied by anterior open bite and delayed eruption of teeth.

HASHIMOTO'S DISEASE (Lymphadenoid goitre)

This is an autoimmune thyroid disease in which antibodies are formed to thyroglobulin and thyroid cells. Chronic inflammation occurs with gradual destruction of the gland. Hypothyroidism results and if untreated may proceed to myxoedema. Treatment is with daily **thyroxine** for life.

Dental Significance

Provided the patients are euthyroid there are no contra-indications to dental treatment and anaesthesia.

GOITRE

Enlargement of the thyroid gland (goitre) may result from hyperthyroidism, or rarely carcinoma, but most commonly as a compensatory response to decrease in circulating thyroid hormone. Decreased thyroid hormone production may result from iodine lack, enzyme defects, antithyroid drugs, and autoimmune or other forms of thyroiditis. Most goitres do not require surgery, the best treatment being reassurance. **Thyroxine** should be tried but significant reduction in gland size is rarely achieved.

Dental Significance

None.

THYROTOXICOSIS, **see THYROID DISEASE.**

TIC DOLOREUX, **see TRIGEMINAL NEURALGIA.**

TINEA

The condition is caused by a fungus, the common sites of infection being:

(1) the scalp (ringworm), where it is seen in children as a circular patch from which the hair has fallen out;
(2) the groin (dhobie itch), where it presents as a red raised butterfly rash which is irritant;
(3) the feet (athlete's foot), where it appears as vesicles and macerated skin between the toes.

The condition is more common in hot weather and frequently picked up in changing-rooms and from infected towels.

Treatment is with topical ointments containing **clotrimazole** (*Canestan*$_{GB}$, *Mycelex*$_{US}$) or **undecenoates** (*Mycota, Tineafax*$_{GB}$) for most infections, but systemic treatment with **griseofulvin** (*Fulcin*$_{GB}$, *Grisovin*$_{GB}$, *Fulvicin*$_{US}$) 125 mg four times daily, will be required if the náils are infected.

Dental Significance

None.

TONSILLITIS

This common disease, characterized by severe sore throat and marked general malaise, occurs predominantly in children and adolescents. The usual organism is a haemolytic streptococcus.

The tonsils are swollen and inflamed with pus exuding from the crypts. Complications include peritonsillar abscess and acute suppurative otitis media.

Symptomatic treatment and **aspirin** or **paracetamol** are usually all that is required. Antibiotics, of which **penicillin V** 250 mg four times daily is the best to start with, should be reserved for follicular tonsillitis and tonsillar abscess (quinsy). A throat swab should be taken and sent for culture and sensitivity assessment.

It should be remembered that tonsillitis is an early feature of many infectious fevers. Tonsillectomy is considered for patients who suffer recurrent attacks of tonsillitis or otitis media.

Dental Significance

Dental treatment should be postponed until the condition has subsided.

TRACHEITIS

Acute tracheitis, together with laryngitis and bronchitis, are frequently the complications of a severe cold or influenza. Their symptoms are well known. Though initially caused by a virus secondary bacterial infection may follow.

Smoking should be avoided and bed-rest and staying indoors is advisable. Inhalations three times a day and at night with **tinct. benz. co.** (5 ml in 500 ml hot water) is helpful, with a cough linctus and analgesics as required.

In the very young, the old, the infirm, and those on immunosuppressive or cytotoxic drugs, antibiotic treatment should be given. **Ampicillin** 6-hourly 250 mg for adults and 12.5 mg/kg for children is probably the best, except for those sensitive to it.

Dental Significance

Patients without severe dental discomfort should be advised to postpone treatment until recovered.

TRIGEMINAL NEURALGIA

The cause of this distressing complaint remains unknown. It is more common in older women and is usually unilateral. The pain, which is severe, occurs in spasms lasting a few seconds to a minute, is precipitated by movement of the mouth or touching the face, and is felt over the distribution area of the maxillary or mandibular division of the trigeminal nerve. Occasionally the condition is associated with multiple sclerosis.

At the present time **carbamazepine** (*Tegretol*$_{GB,US}$) is the treatment of choice, starting with a dose of 50 mg three times daily and increasing until the symptoms disappear or unpleasant side-effects such as dizziness or skin rashes occur (usually 200 mg three times daily). Various surgical procedures, which include destruction or division of the nerve or ganglion, are available for those who are not helped by drug therapy, but their disadvantages need carefully explaining before they are undertaken. More recently vascular surgery to a loop of the cerebellar artery pressing on the nerve root has claimed a high success rate without unpleasant sequelae.

Dental Significance

As the trigger point may be in or around the mouth, and spasm provoked by cleaning the teeth, bad oral hygiene is not uncommon and patients may be very reluctant to submit to dental examination.

Intermittent attacks of acute pulpitis or pain from a damaged inferior dental nerve may cause similar symptoms, and must be considered in the differential diagnosis.

TUBERCULOSIS

Though much less common than it used to be, tuberculosis is still seen widely in this country, causing significant morbidity and mortality. Any system in the body can be involved so presentation may be extremely variable and diagnosis often very difficult. Two strains of **Mycobacterium tuberculosis,** human and bovine, cause disease in man.

Infection may be localized to the skin, lungs, gastrointestinal tract, kidneys, bones, lymph glands, liver, adrenals, meninges, or joints and symptoms are those of the involved system. When infected material enters the circulation, generalized disease results leading to miliary tuberculosis. This occurs in people with chronic tuberculosis or in the immunosuppressed. Symptoms become generalized and include fatigue, headache, weight loss, night sweats, and fever.

The diagnosis is suspected by characteristic radiological or clinical findings and confirmed by demonstrating the bacillus in tissue or body secretions and growing it in culture or in guinea-pigs. The disadvantage of the latter method is the delay of 4 or more weeks waiting for the result.

The incidence of tuberculosis has been greatly reduced by the introduction of the BCG vaccine (bacillus Calmette–Guérin), an attenuated strain of the tubercle bacillus. The Mantoux or Heaf skin test is used to assess immune status and if negative the vaccine is given. Vaccine should be offered to children from 10–13 years and to all immigrants.

The prognosis of tuberculosis has been radically altered by the refinement of antituberculous antibiotics. Treatment has two phases: an initial phase when at least three drugs are used for 8 weeks or more, and a continuation phase when the drugs are reduced to two for 9 months. Drugs of choice are **isoniazid** (up to 300 mg daily), **rifampicin** (450–600 mg daily), and **ethambutol** (*Mynah*$_{GB}$, Myambutol$_{GB,US}$) (15 mg/kg daily).

Dental Significance

Tuberculous ulcers occur in the mouth, more commonly on the tongue, and are usually secondary to pulmonary infection. They have a ragged outline and are generally painful. The bacilli are too scanty to be identified from a smear, and biopsy and culture are required. Patients with suspected tuberculous ulcers should be referred to their doctor for general assessment.

Tuberculous infection of the cervical lymph glands is now less common. Initially the swollen gland is painful and discrete but later becomes bound to the skin and may discharge through a sinus.

Tuberculosis of the salivary glands, and tuberculous osteomyelitis of the mandible, are fortunately rare.

Early diagnosis and treatment are important components in the fight against TB and dentists should remain alert to signs of the disease in the head and neck, especially amongst recent immigrants.

TUBEROUS SCLEROSIS (Epiloia)

This is a neurocutaneous disorder inherited as an autosomal dominant trait and characterized by facial naevi (adenoma sebaceum), epilepsy, and mental retardation.

Dental Significance

The hyperplasia of the sebaceous glands (adenoma sebaceum) frequently affects the lower lip.

TYPHOID FEVER (Enteric Fever)

Typhoid results from infection by *Salmonella typhi*, a Gram-negative rod, and occurs in areas of poor hygiene or where food or drinking water has become contaminated by human sewage. It is primarily a bacteraemic illness with abdominal symptoms occurring at some stage. The organism is swallowed and crosses the gut to multiply in mesenteric glands before disseminating. The incubation period is 10–14 days. The severity of the illness varies and may be no more than a mild transitory illness. However, classically during the first week the symptoms are of malaise, lethargy, headache, fever, and anorexia. The characteristic rose spots, 2–4 mm in diameter, occur in only 10–20 per cent of cases. During the second week there is a persistent pyrexia, tachycardia, delirium, distended abdomen, diarrhoea, and splenomegaly. During the third week the temperature usually settles but in a small proportion the disease progresses with severe toxicity, coma, and occasionally bowel perforation or haemorrhage. Early diagnosis and treatment with **chloramphenicol** (1 g 6-hourly for 7 days) or **ampicillin** (1 g 4-hourly) prevents the natural progression of the disease. Active immunization with two injections of Vaccine (TAB) 4 weeks apart, or monovalent typhoid vaccine, is an essential part of preventative treatment.

Dental Significance

Parotitis is an unpleasant complication of the disease and the dentist should be ready to advise on oral hygiene to help to avoid this.

U

ULCERATIVE COLITIS, see COLITIS.

UNDULANT FEVER, see BRUCELLOSIS.

URAEMIA, see RENAL DISEASE.

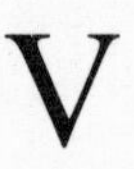

VARICELLA (Chicken pox)

Though more common in childhood, adults may catch the infection, when it tends to be more severe. The causative virus is the same as that of herpes zoster, and children may pick up chicken pox from an adult with shingles, but not the other way round.

The usual incubation period is 15–18 days and the condition frequently starts with general malaise and a prodomal erythematous rash. The characteristic vesicles appear first on the head and trunk and spread outwards.

As yet there is no vaccine against varicella and treatment is symptomatic with mild analgesics and **lotio calamine** and/or **trimeprazine** (*Vallergan*$_{GB}$) (*Temaril*$_{US}$) to reduce the irritation. With immuno-deficiency the infection may be severe and intravenous **acyclovar** is proving helpful.

Dental Significance

Vesicles may occur in the mouth, more commonly on the palate or fauces. They quickly break down to small ulcers with a surrounding area of erythema, which cause little discomfort and no treatment is required.

Dentists should appreciate the infectivity of the condition particularly in the early stages and/or with lesions in the mouth, and prevent suspected cases coming in contact with other children. After examination instruments and the rinse-out glass should be thoroughly sterilized.

VASCULAR DISEASE

ARTERIAL ANEURYSM

An aneurysm is a permanent dilatation of an artery due to destruction of its wall. It may be congenital, traumatic, inflammatory, or degenerative.

Congenital aneurysms are confined to the base of the brain in the circle of Willis. The so-called 'Berry' aneurysm results from a defect of the media. Rupture leads to subarachnoid haemorrhage (see INTRACRANIAL HAEMORRHAGE).

Traumatic aneurysms result from penetrating injuries such as gunshot wounds.

Inflammation due to such diseases as syphilis, bacterial endocarditis, and polyarteritis nodosum may cause aneurysms. Syphilis affects the aorta. Mycotic aneurysms result from infected emboli and are seen in subacute bacterial endocarditis.

Atheroma is the commonest degenerative lesion causing aneurysm formation. The aorta may be affected at any site but most commonly in the abdomen below the renal arteries. Pain or awareness of abdominal pulsation are the most frequent symptoms although commonly no symptoms precede aneurysmal rupture. An aneurysm may be a chance finding on examination. Complications include rupture, thrombosis, and embolism. Treatment when possible is surgical.

Dental Significance

As for atheroma.

ATHEROMA

This is the commonest form of arterial degeneration. It is a generalized disease increasing with age, affecting particularly the arteries of the heart, brain, kidneys, and limbs. Arterial narrowing results from a combination of atheromatous plaque formation and internal thrombosis. It may result in progressive impairment of blood supply. In the coronary arteries this causes angina and infarction; in the kidneys renal failure; in the cerebral arteries dementia, and cerebrovascular accidents; and in the legs claudication, ischaemia, and gangrene.

The cause of atheroma is obscure but high cholesterol level, high intake of saturated animal fats, hypertension, and diabetes are all important factors in its development.

Dental Significance

Because of their abundant blood supply, structures of the mouth are seldom affected by atheroma, though it may be found in the arteries supplying them.

Sometimes the pain of angina pectoris may be referred to the mouth or throat and suggest an oral pathology.

Patients with atheroma can be offered the full scope of dental treatment, but aspirating syringes and local anaesthetic without **adrenaline** should always be used. The hazard of general anaesthetics is increased in patients with the condition, but it can be justifiably claimed that, in a nervous patient, the anxiety of a dental extraction with local anaesthesia can be equally damaging. Providing the atheromatous condition is not advanced, short general anaesthetics can be given in the surgery making sure that anaesthetic gases always contain 50 per cent oxygen.

STROKE

Cerebral thrombosis, haemorrhage, and embolism lead to brain damage and infarction of the area of the brain supplied by the [illegible]luded vessel or damaged by the haemorrhage. The resulting neurological deficit, which may vary from minimal impairment of function to gross paralysis, is termed a stroke or cerebrovascular accident.

Cerebral atheroma and hypertension are major factors underlying strokes. Thromboses are commoner than haemorrhages, which are more often rapidly fatal. The commonest site for both is in the territory of the middle cerebral artery in the internal capsule.

In the carotid system the most common feature is a hemiplegia often accompanied by visual impairment and, if in the dominant hemisphere, impairment of speech as well. The vertebral system, when involved, may give rise to a mixture of signs. Damage to long tracts causes hemiplegia, but in addition damage to brain stem, cranial nerve nuclei, and their tracts results in a variety of cranial nerve defects and damage to cerebellar pathways causing ataxia.

Management is aimed at carefully graded rehabilitation with close co-operation between doctor, physiotherapist, occupational therapist, and nurse. There is little place for anticoagulants. Hypertension should be treated but not too precipitously.

Occasionally the neurological signs of a stroke are fleeting and disappear. Such an event is termed a transient ischaemic episode. In the majority of patients with such attacks a definitive stroke usually occurs within a year. It is therefore important to consider further investigations in this group in an attempt to find treatable lesions and prevent further strokes occurring. These patients may be helped by low-dose **aspirin** (300 mg daily).

Dental Significance

Advice and assistance with oral hygiene is important if paralysis involves structures of the mouth. Conservation of the natural dentition is advisable as these patients frequently have trouble managing dentures. It is wise to use local anaesthetics without **adrenaline** and administer general anaesthetics in hospital.

VITAMIN DEFICIENCIES

VITAMIN A (RETINOL)

Vitamin A is present in green vegetables, milk, and animal fats. Deficiency, which is seldom seen in Great Britain, causes xerophthalmia, conjunctival ulceration, and night-blindness.

Dental Significance

Xerostomia and keratinization in the mouth have been observed in vitamin A deficiency.

VITAMIN B1 (THIAMINE)

Deficiency causes beri-beri, a disease uncommon in the UK but sometimes seen in alcoholics. Symptoms include polyneuritis, muscle weakness, encephalopathy (Wernicke's encephalopathy), and cardiac failure. No oral manifestations are known.

VITAMIN B2 (RIBOFLAVINE)

Deficiency results in changes in the skin and mucous membranes. Seborrhoeic dermatitis, a bright red tongue, and angular cheilitis are the common symptoms. Vascularization of the cornea occurs and is a diagnostic point. Treatment by taking brewers' yeast or vitamin B2, 10 mg daily, corrects the deficiency.

VITAMIN B6 (PYRIDOXINE)

Deficiency is rare but has been reported in patients with tuberculosis being treated with **isoniazid**. Muscle weakness, neuritis, and stomato-glossitis are the common symptoms. Deficiency should be corrected by taking pyridoxine 30–60 mg daily.

NICOTINIC ACID

Deficiency, not normally seen in the UK, causes pellagra, whose features include dermatitis, erythema of the mucosa with papillary atrophy of the tongue, together with neurological disorders.

VITAMIN B12

The daily requirement of this vitamin, found only in animal products, is very small indeed and signs of deficiency usually result from a failure to absorb it. The clinical picture and oral manifestations are described under the heading of ANAEMIA (PERNICIOUS ANAEMIA).

FOLIC ACID

Folic acid is present in yeast, green vegetables, and animal products. The body requirements are small but deficiency can occur in pregnant women, alcoholics, the old, and the debilitated. Certain lesions of the alimentary tract such as coeliac and Crohn's disease can interfere with its absorption, and various drugs act as antagonists, notably **methotrexate** (a cytotoxic drug), **trimethoprim** (an antibacterial), and most anticonvulsant drugs (**phenobarbitone** and **phenytoin**).

The clinical picture produced by folic acid deficiency is identical to that of pernicious anaemia except for the neurological features which complicate vitamin B12 deficiency (see SUBACUTE COMBINED DEGENERATION OF THE CORD), and the differential diagnosis can only be made by micro-biological and radio-assay tests.

Oral administration of folic acid in a dosage of 5 mg three times daily corrects the deficiency but should be administered with care as it has a potential hazard of exacerbating subacute combined degeneration of the cord in undiagnosed vitamin B12 deficiency.

Dental Significance

The deficiency should be borne in mind in the class of patients susceptible, when the dentist is presented with a 'raw beef' tongue, recurrent mouth ulcers, and angular cheilitis.

VITAMIN C (ASCORBIC ACID)

Deficiency of vitamin C, the vitamin of citrus fruit and fresh vegetables, leads to scurvy with swelling and ulceration of the gums and bleeding at the gingival margin. The diagnosis is confirmed by assaying the leucocyte vitamin C concentration, a reading of less than 10 $\mu g/10^6$ cells being positive.

Overt clinical scurvy is now rare in Great Britain, but recent research has shown that up to 50 per cent of the elderly and debilitated have leucocyte levels of vitamin C down to scurvy level in the winter months. Vitamin C is important in the synthesis of collagen, and as such plays a part in healing of wounds; but other properties, such as stimulating leucocyte function and aiding immune responses, remain unproven.

Vitamin C, taken by mouth in a daily dosage of 100 mg, is sufficient to correct any deficiency. Higher dosage appears harmless but unnecessary.

Dental Significance

Gingival inflammation of the elderly during the winter months should raise suspicions of vitamin C deficiency, and, as vitamin C supplement is simple and harmless, it should be prescribed if no other pathology is obvious.

VITAMIN D (CHOLECALCIFEROL)

Deficiency of vitamin D causes rickets in the young and osteomalacia in adults. Its main dietary sources are eggs, butter, milk, and fish-liver oils. It is also formed in the skin under the influence of sunlight. The symptoms of rickets are painful swellings at the ends of the long bones and ribs (rickety rosary), fronto-parietal bosses on the skull, and muscle weakness. Severe bone pain is a characteristic of osteomalacia, especially at the sites of pseudofractures (Looser's zone).

The condition is seen in the UK more commonly in Asian immigrants, the elderly and housebound, and those on treatment with anticonvulsants or **aluminium hydroxide**.

Renal rickets results from failure in renal metabolism of vitamin D.

Treatment is with vitamin D, 2000 units daily in dietary insufficiency. For renal rickets and hypoparathyroidism very large doses (50,000–150,000 units per day) are required.

Dental Significance

Surprisingly, the teeth are little affected and enamel hypoplasia is rare. X-rays may show elongation of the pulp horns and in the mandible and maxilla there is diminished thickness of cortical bone and the lamina dura.

VITAMIN E

Except perhaps in premature infants, there is doubt about the necessity of this substance. No oral manifestations of deficiency have been recorded.

VITAMINS K1 AND K2

Vitamin K1 is found in green vegetables and vitamin K2 is synthesized by bacteria in the intestine. Together they are essential for the synthesis of various factors in clotting of the blood.

Deficiency usually results from either a sterile gut, as in the newborn, or from malabsorption as a result of obstructive jaundice or steatorrhoea, particularly in the face of oral antibiotic therapy. Anticoagulants act competitively with vitamin K and prevent the synthesis of clotting factors.

Where there is deficiency, vitamin K is best given by intramuscular injection (10–20 mg).

Dental Significance

Patients with conditions which predispose to vitamin K deficiency are at risk with surgery or extractions, and should be given vitamin K supplement 6–8 hours prior to operation.

VON RECKLINGHAUSEN'S DISEASE, **see** NEUROFIBROMATOSIS.

VON WILLEBRAND'S DISEASE, **see** HAEMOPHILIA.

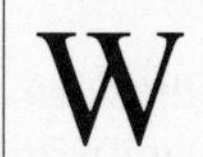

WALDENSTROM'S MACROGLOBULINAEMIA, see MACROGLOBULINAEMIA.

WATERHOUSE–FRIDERICHSEN SYNDROME (Fulminating meningococcal septicaemia)

This is an overwhelming septicaemic illness associated with haemorrhages into the adrenal cortices and elsewhere, in which death is usual within 4–24 hours of onset. It most commonly occurs in young children. If the diagnosis can be made early enough, life can be saved.

Dental Significance

None.

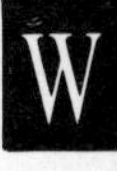

WEGENER'S GRANULOMA

This is probably a variant of polyarteritis nodosum, characterized by ulcerating nasal granulomata and necrotic lesions in the lung. It occurs in middle life, equally in both sexes, and is accompanied by fever, cough, haemoptysis, and pleurisy. Prognosis is poor but may be improved by treatment with corticosteroids.

Dental Significance

The condition also involves the mouth, where it takes the form of granulomatous swelling of the interdental papillae with destruction of the alveolus below. Extraction sockets display the same picture and fail to heal properly.

WEIL'S DISEASE, see LEPTOSPIROSIS.

WERNICKE'S ENCEPHALOPATHY, see VITAMIN DEFICIENCIES. (Vitamin B1).

WHIPPLE'S DISEASE

This rare disorder, predominantly of middle-aged men, is characterized by malabsorption, arthritis, and lymphadenopathy. Diagnosis is made by jejunal biopsy demonstrating distortion of mucosal anatomy by large quantities of periodic acid Schiff (PAS) material in the lamina propria. This is the end-product of bacterial degradation and a small rod-shaped organism has been demonstrated in the mucosa. The condition responds well to **tetracycline** (250 mg four times a day for 2 years).

Dental Significance

None.

WHOOPING COUGH, see PERTUSSIS.

WILSON'S DISEASE, see LIVER DISEASE.

WOLFF–PARKINSON–WHITE SYNDROME, see HEART DISEASE (Congenital).

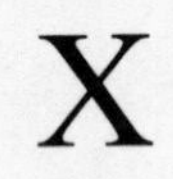

XANTHOMATOSES, see **HYPERLIPIDAEMIA.**

Z

ZOLLINGER–ELLISON SYNDROME

The symptoms of this condition result from excessive gastric acid secretion due to non-B cell adenoma or islet cell hyperplasia of the pancreas producing abnormal quantities of gastrin. Abnormal and extensive peptic ulceration occurs extending into the second part of the duodenum. Diarrhoea, bleeding, and perforation are complications. Diagnosis is confirmed by grossly raised serum gastrin levels and treatment, where possible, is excision of the tumour and gastrectomy. Where surgery is not possible medical control with H2 receptor antagonists, **cimetidine** (*Tagamet*$_{GB,US}$) or **ranitidine** (*Zantac*$_{GB}$) has been very successful.

Dental Significance

As for PEPTIC ULCER.

ZOSTER, see HERPES ZOSTER.

X Z

SECTION 2

Alphabetical List of Pharmacological and Proprietary Drug Names

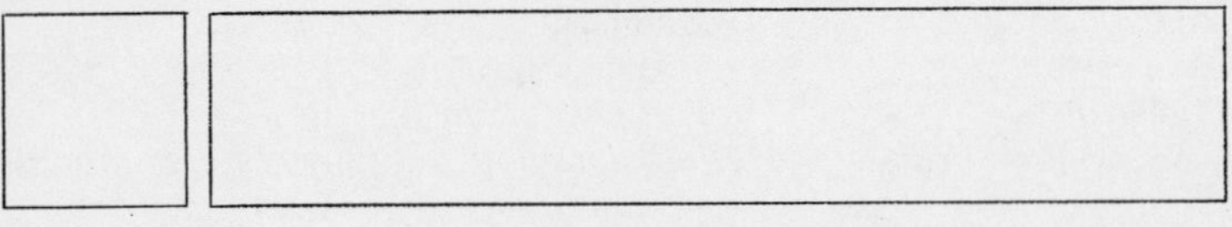

Abidec$_{GB}$	multivitamin preparation
Acebutolol$_{GB}$	(*Sectral*$_{GB}$), a beta-blocker
Acetazolamide$_{GB,US}$	(*Diamox*$_{GB,US}$), carbonic anhydrase inhibitor used in glaucoma
Acetohexamide$_{GB\ US}$	(*Dimelor*$_{GB}$), hypoglycaemic agent
achromycin$_{GB,US}$	see **tetracycline**$_{GB,US}$
actal$_{GB}$	antacid
acthar$_{GB,US}$	see **corticotrophin**$_{GB}$
actifed$_{GB,US}$	cough compound
Actinomycin$_{GB}$	cytotoxic antibiotic, main use in childhood solid tumours, causes marrow depression
actrapid$_{GB,US}$	see **insulin**$_{GB,US}$
acupan$_{GB}$	see **nefopam**$_{GB}$
Acyclovir$_{GB}$	(*Zovirax*$_{GB}$) antiviral preparation
adalat$_{GB}$	see **nifedipine**$_{GB}$
adcortyl$_{GB}$	see **triamcinolone**$_{GB,US}$
Adrenocorticotrophic hormone$_{GB,US}$	see **corticotrophin**$_{GB}$
adriamycin$_{GB,US}$	see **doxorubicin hydrochloride**$_{GB,US}$
albucid$_{GB}$	see **sulphacetamide**$_{GB,US}$
aldactide$_{GB}$	**spironolactone**$_{GB,US}$ + **hydroflumethiazide**$_{GB,US}$
aldactone$_{GB,US}$	see **spironolactone**$_{GB,US}$
aldomet$_{GB,US}$	see **methyldopa**$_{GB,US}$
alkeran$_{GB,US}$	see **melphalan**$_{GB,US}$
Allopurinol$_{GB,US}$	(*Zyloric*$_{GB}$, *Zyloprim*$_{US}$, *Lopurin*$_{US}$), xanthine oxidase inhibitor for treatment of hyperuricaemia
Altacite$_{GB}$	see **hydrotalcite**$_{GB}$
Aludrox$_{GB,US}$	see **aluminium hydroxide**$_{GB,US}$
Aluminium hydroxide$_{GB,US}$	antacid
Alupent$_{GB,US}$	see **orciprenaline**$_{GB}$
Amantadine$_{GB,US}$	(*Symmetrel*$_{GB,US}$), dopaminergic drug used in Parkinsonism

Amcill$_{US}$	see **ampicillin**$_{GB,US}$
Amicar$_{US}$	see **Aminocaproic acid**$_{GB,US}$
Amiloride$_{GB}$	potassium-sparing diuretic
Aminocaproic acid$_{GB,US}$	(*Epsikapron*$_{GB}$), antifibrinolytic drug used for haemorrhage after surgery
Aminophylline$_{GB,US}$	xanthine derivative used in asthma
Amitid$_{US}$	see **amitriptyline**$_{GB,US}$
Amitriptyline$_{GB,US}$	(*Amitid*$_{US}$), tricyclic antidepressant, causes a dry mouth, use LAs without **adrenaline**
Amoxil$_{GB,US}$	see **amoxycillin**$_{GB,US}$
amoxycillin$_{GB,US}$	ampicillin derivative with similar antibacterial spectrum but twice as well absorbed by mouth
Amphetamine$_{GB,US}$	central nervous stimulant—its use may lead to dependence and psychotic states
Amphotericin$_{GB,US}$	(*Fungilin*$_{GB}$, *Fungizone*$_{GB,US}$), anti-fungal drug which can be given systemically
Ampicillin$_{GB,US}$	(*Penbritin*$_{GB}$, *Amcill*$_{US}$), antibiotic active against certain Gram-positive and Gram-negative organisms but inactivated by penicillinases, may affect the absorption of oral contraceptives
Ampiclox$_{GB}$	**Ampicillin**$_{GB,US}$ + **Cloxicillin**$_{GB,US}$
Amylobarbitone$_{GB}$	a hypnotic and sedative—little used now
Amytal$_{GB,US}$	see **amylobarbitone**$_{GB}$
Anafranil$_{GB}$	see **clomipramine**$_{GB}$
Andursil$_{GB}$	antacid mixture
Antabuse$_{GB,US}$	see **disulfiram**$_{GB,US}$
Antepar$_{GB,US}$	see **piperazine**$_{GB,US}$
Anturan$_{GB,US}$	see **sulphinpyrazone**$_{GB,US}$
Apresoline$_{GB,US}$	see **hydralazine**$_{GB,US}$
Aprinox$_{GB}$	see **bendrofluazide**$_{GB}$
Aprotinin$_{GB}$	(*Trasylol*$_{GB}$), a proteolytic enzyme inhibitor used in acute pancreatitis
Aralen$_{US}$	see **chloroquine**$_{GB,US}$
Artane$_{GB,US}$	see **benzhexol**$_{GB,US}$
Asilone$_{GB}$	antacid mixture
Aspirin$_{GB,US}$	analgesic, potentiates action of **warfarin** and oral hypoglycaemics
Atenolol$_{GB}$	beta-blocker, hypotensive effect of general anaesthetics potentiated
Ativan$_{GB,US}$	see **lorazepam**$_{GB,US}$

Atromid$_{\text{GB,US}}$	see **clofibrate**$_{\text{GB,US}}$
Atropine$_{\text{GB,US}}$	anticholinergic drug, not to be given to patients with glaucoma
Atrovent$_{\text{GB}}$	see **ipratropium bromide**$_{\text{GB}}$
Aureocort$_{\text{GB}}$	compound skin preparation
Aureomycin$_{\text{GB,US}}$	see **chlortetracycline**$_{\text{GB,US}}$
Avloclor$_{\text{GB}}$	see **chloroquine**$_{\text{GB,US}}$
Avomine$_{\text{GB}}$	see **promethazine theoclate**$_{\text{GB,US}}$
Azapropazone$_{\text{GB}}$	(*Rheumox*$_{\text{GB}}$), non-steroidal anti-inflammatory drug
Azathioprine$_{\text{GB,US}}$	(*Imuran*$_{\text{GB,US}}$), immunosuppressant agent, used to prevent transplant rejection and in certain other conditions, collagen disorders, and Crohn's disease, may cause marrow depression
Azulfidine$_{\text{US}}$	see **sulphasalazine**$_{\text{GB,US}}$
Baclofen$_{\text{GB,US}}$	(*Lioresal*$_{\text{GB,US}}$), muscle relaxant; used for muscle spasm in spastic conditions
Bactrim$_{\text{GB,US}}$	see **co-trimoxazole**$_{\text{GB,US}}$
Beclomethasone$_{\text{GB,US}}$	(*Becotide*$_{\text{GB}}$, *Beclovent*$_{\text{US}}$), *corticosteroid used in aerosol inhalation or insufflation form for bronchospasm, occasionally suppresses adrenals*
Beclovent$_{\text{US}}$	see **beclomethasone**$_{\text{GB,US}}$
Beconase$_{\text{GB}}$	see **beclomethasone**$_{\text{GB,US}}$
Becotide$_{\text{GB}}$	see **beclomethasone**$_{\text{GB,US}}$
Belladonna$_{\text{GB,US}}$	anticholinergic agent, may cause a dry mouth
Bellergal$_{\text{GB,US}}$	mixture: **phenobarbitone**$_{\text{GB,US}}$, **belladonna**$_{\text{GB,US}}$, **ergotamine**$_{\text{GB,US}}$
Benadryl$_{\text{GB,US}}$	see **diphenhydramine**$_{\text{GB,US}}$
Bendrofluazide$_{\text{GB}}$	thiazide diuretic
Benemid$_{\text{GB,US}}$	see **probenecid**$_{\text{GB,US}}$
Benoral$_{\text{GB}}$	see **benorylate**$_{\text{GB}}$
Benorylate$_{\text{GB}}$	non-steroidal, anti-inflammatory agent
Benoxaprofen$_{\text{GB}}$	non-steroidal, anti-inflammatory agent
Benserazide$_{\text{GB}}$	(with **levodopa in** *Madopar*$_{\text{GB}}$), extracerebral dopa-decarboxylase inhibitor for Parkinsonism
Benzedrine$_{\text{US}}$	see **amphetamine**$_{\text{GB,US}}$

Benzehexol$_{GB}$	(*Artane*$_{GB,US}$), anticholinergic drug used in Parkinsonism
Benzodiazepines	hypnotic, sedative, and anxiolylic drugs
Benzyl benzoate$_{GB}$	*Ascabiol*$_{GB}$, treatment of scabies
Beta-cardone$_{GB}$	see **sotalol**$_{GB}$
Betahistine hydrochloride$_{GB}$	*Serc*$_{GB}$, for vertigo and hearing disturbances in labyrinthine disorders
Betaloc$_{GB}$	see **metoprolol**$_{GB,US}$
Betamethasone$_{GB,US}$	corticosteroid with little mineralocorticoid action, useful in certain dermatological disorders, may suppress adrenals
Bethanidine$_{GB}$	(*Esbatal*$_{GB}$), adrenergic neurone-blocking hypotensive agent, can cause discomfort in salivary glands, potentiates hypotensive effect of general anaesthetics
Betnovate$_{GB}$	compound skin preparation
Bextasol$_{GB}$	see **betamethasone valerate**$_{GB,US}$
Biogastrone$_{GB}$	see **carbenoxolone sodium**$_{GB}$
Bisacodyl$_{GB,US}$	powerful stimulant laxative (*Dulcolax*$_{GB,US}$)
Bisolvon$_{GB}$	see **bromhexine**$_{GB}$
Blenoxane$_{US}$	see **bleomycin**$_{GB,US}$
Bleomycin$_{GB,US}$	cytotoxic agent (*Blenoxane*$_{US}$), causes marrow suppression
Blocadren$_{GB}$	see **timolol**$_{GB,US}$
Bolvidon$_{GB}$	see **mianserin**$_{GB}$
Bonjela$_{GB}$	see **choline salicylate**$_{GB,US}$
Bricanyl$_{GB,US}$	see **terbutaline**$_{GB,US}$
Bromhexine$_{GB}$	mucolytic agent (*Bisolvon*$_{GB}$)
Bromocriptine$_{GB,US}$	stimulates dopamine receptors (used in Parkinsonism) (*Parlodel*$_{GB,US}$)
Brufen$_{GB,US}$	see **ibuprofen**$_{GB,US}$
Buclizine hydrochloride$_{GB,US}$	(in *Migraleve*$_{GB}$), treatment for migraine
Bumetanide$_{GB}$	loop diuretic (*Burinex*$_{GB}$)
Buprenorphine$_{GB}$	powerful analgesic (*Temgesic*$_{GB}$), not to be used on patients taking MAOIs
Burinex$_{GB}$	see **bumetanide**$_{GB}$
Buscopan$_{GB}$	see **hyoscine**$_{GB,US}$
Busulphan$_{GB,US}$	cytotoxic agent (*Myleran*$_{GB,US}$), causes marrow depression
Butacote$_{GB}$	see **phenylbutazone**$_{GB,US}$
Butazolidine$_{GB,US}$	see **phenylbutazone**$_{GB,US}$

Butabarbital$_{US}$ } barbiturate (*Soneryl*$_{GB}$)
Butabarbitone$_{GB}$ }

Cafergot$_{GB,US}$ see **ergotamine tartrate**$_{GB,US}$

Caladryl$_{GB,US}$ compound skin preparation

Calamine$_{GB,US}$ local anti-pruritic agent (*Caladryl*$_{GB,US}$)

Calciferol$_{GB,US}$ vitamin D

Calcimar$_{US}$ see **calcitonin**$_{GB,US}$

Calcitare$_{GB}$ see **calcitonin**$_{GB}$

Calcitonin$_{GB,US}$ (*Calcitare*$_{GB}$, *Calcimar*$_{US}$), lowers serum calcium level—used in Paget's disease and hyperparathyroidism

Canesten Cream$_{GB}$ see **clotrimazole**$_{GB,US}$

Capoten$_{GB}$ see **captopril**

Captopril$_{GB}$ used in treatment of severe hypertensions. Loss of taste and a scalding sensation in the mouth have been reported. General anaesthetic to be avoided

Carbachol$_{GB}$ mydriatic

Carbamazepine$_{GB,US}$ anti-epileptic and used in trigeminal neuralgia (*Tegretol*$_{GB,US}$), reduces effect of oral contraceptives and anticoagulants and not to be given within 2 weeks of MAOIs

Carbenicillin$_{GB,US}$ anti-pseudomonal penicillin (*Pyopen*$_{GB,US}$)

Carbenoxolone sodium$_{GB}$ (*Biogastrone, Duogastrone*) for peptic ulcer healing

Carbidopa$_{GB,US}$ (*Sinemet*$_{GB,US}$), dopaminergic drug for Parkinsonism, avoid use of **halothane**

Carbimazole$_{GB}$ antithyroid drug

Catapres$_{GB,US}$ see **clonidine**$_{GB,US}$

Caved-S$_{GB}$ deglycyrrhizinized liquorice

CCNU$_{GB}$ see **lomustine**$_{GB,US}$

Cefoxitin$_{GB,US}$ cephalosporin antibiotic (*Mefoxin*$_{GB,US}$)

Cefuroxime$_{GB}$ cephalosporin antibiotic (*Zinacef*$_{GB}$)

Celevac$_{GB}$ see **methylcellulose**$_{GB,US}$

Cephalexin$_{GB,US}$ cephalosporin antibiotic (*Ceporex*$_{GB}$, *Keflex*$_{GB,US}$)

Cephaloridine$_{GB,US}$ (*Ceporin*$_{GB}$), cephalosporin antibiotic (*Loridine*$_{US}$)

Cephalothin$_{GB,US}$ (*Keflin*$_{GB,US}$), cephalosporin antibiotic

Cephazolin$_{\text{GB}}$	(*Kefzol*$_{\text{GB,US}}$), cephalosporin antibiotic
Cephradine$_{\text{GB,US}}$	(*Velosef*$_{\text{GB,US}}$), cephalosporin antibiotic
Ceporex$_{\text{GB}}$	see **cephalexin**$_{\text{GB,US}}$
Ceporin$_{\text{GB}}$	see **cephaloridine**$_{\text{GB,US}}$
Cetiprin$_{\text{GB}}$	see **emepronium bromide**$_{\text{GB}}$
Chenodeoxycholic acid$_{\text{GB}}$	(*Chendol*), gallstone dissolving agent
Chloral$_{\text{GB,US}}$	hypnotic and sedative
Chlorambucil$_{\text{GB,US}}$	(*Leukeran*$_{\text{GB,US}}$), alkylating cytotoxic drug causes marrow depression
Chloramphenicol$_{\text{GB,US}}$	(*Chloromycetin*$_{\text{GB,US}}$, *Kemicetine*$_{\text{GB}}$), antibiotic
Chlordiazepoxide$_{\text{GB,US}}$	(*Librium*$_{\text{GB,US}}$), anxiolytic agent
Chlorhexidine$_{\text{GB,US}}$	(*Corsodyl*$_{\text{GB}}$), mouthwash, gargle, and dentifrice
Chlormethiazole$_{\text{GB}}$	(*Heminevrin*$_{\text{GB}}$), hypnotic and sedative
Chloromycetin$_{\text{GB,US}}$	see **chloramphenicol**$_{\text{GB,US}}$
Chloroquine$_{\text{US GB}}$	(*Aralen*$_{\text{US}}$, *Avloclor*$_{\text{GB}}$), antimalarial agent, can cause oral erosions
Chlorothiazide$_{\text{US GB}}$	thiazide diuretic
Chlorpheniramine$_{\text{US GB}}$	(*Piriton*$_{\text{GB}}$), antihistamine
Chlorpromazine$_{\text{US GB}}$	(*Largactil*$_{\text{GB}}$), antipsychotic drug, hypotensive effect of general anaesthetics potentiated
Chlorpropamide$_{\text{US GB}}$	(*Diabinese*$_{\text{GB,US}}$), hypoglycaemic agent, potentiated by **aspirin**, can cause oral erosions
Chlortetracycline$_{\text{US GB}}$	antibiotic
Chlorthalidone$_{\text{GB,US}}$	(*Hygroton*$_{\text{GB,US}}$), diuretic
Cholecalciferol$_{\text{GB}}$	vitamin D
Choledyl$_{\text{GB,US}}$	see **choline theophyllinate**$_{\text{GB}}$
Cholestyramine$_{\text{GB,US}}$	(*Questran*$_{\text{GB,US}}$). ion-exchange resin used in hyperlipidaemia and liver disease
Choline salicylate$_{\text{GB,US}}$	(*Bonjela*$_{\text{GB}}$) pain relief in mouth ulceration
Choline theophyllinate$_{\text{GB}}$	(*Choledyl*$_{\text{GB}}$), bronchodilator
Cimetidine$_{\text{GB,US}}$	(*Tagamet*$_{\text{GB,US}}$), H2 receptor antagonist used for treatment of peptic ulcers; effect of **diazepam** is extended, absorption of **tetracyclines** reduced
Cinnarizine$_{\text{GB}}$	(*Stugeron*$_{\text{GB}}$), used for nausea and vomiting
Cleocin$_{\text{US}}$	*see* **clindamycin**$_{\text{GB,US}}$

Clindamycin$_{GB,US}$	(*Cleocin*$_{US}$, *Dalacin C*$_{GB}$), antibiotic, may cause pseudomembranous colitis
Clinoril$_{GB,US}$	see **sulindac**$_{GB,US}$
Clobetasol proprionate$_{GB}$	(*Dermovate*$_{GB}$), topical steroid
Clofibrate$_{GB,US}$	(*Atromid*$_{GB,US}$), for hyperlipidaemia
Clomiphene$_{GB,US}$	(*Clomid*$_{GB,US}$), an anti-oestrogen for inducing ovulation
Clomipramine$_{GB}$	(*Anafranil*$_{GB}$), tricyclic anti-depressant, use LAs without **adrenaline**
Clonazepam$_{GB,US}$	(*Rivotril*$_{GB}$), (*Clonopin*$_{US}$), for epilepsy and myoclonic jerks
Clonidine$_{GB,US}$	(*Catapres*$_{GB,US}$, *Dixarit*$_{GB}$), hypotensive agent, may cause discomfort in salivary glands
Clonopin$_{US}$	see **clonazepam**$_{GB,US}$
Clorazepate dipotassium$_{US,GB}$	(*Tranxene*$_{GB,US}$), anxiolytic agent, *Canesten*$_{GB}$
Clotrimazole$_{US,GB}$	(*Mycelex*$_{US}$), antifungal agent
Cloxacillin$_{GB,US}$	(*Tegopen*$_{US}$), antibiotic used for infections due to penicillinase-producing staphylococci
Co-betaloc$_{GB}$	see **metoprolol**$_{GB,US}$
Co-dergocrine mesylate$_{GB}$	(*Hydergine*$_{GB,US}$), cerebral vasodilator
Cocaine$_{GB}$	an addictive drug causing central nervous stimulation
Codeine phosphate$_{GB,US}$	analgesic, anti-diarrhoeal agent
Codis$_{GB}$	**Aspirin**$_{GB,US}$ + **codeine phosphate**$_{GB,US}$
Colchicine$_{US,GB}$	used in acute gout
Colistin$_{US,GB}$	a polymyxin antibiotic used against Gram-negative organisms
Colofac$_{GB}$	see **mebeverine**$_{GB}$
Compazine$_{US}$	see **prochlorperazine**$_{US}$
Concordin$_{GB}$	see **protriptyline**$_{GB,US}$
Cordilox$_{GB}$	see **verapamil**$_{GB}$
Corgard$_{GB,US}$	see **nadolol**$_{GB,US}$
Corsodyl$_{GB}$	see **chlorhexidine**$_{GB,US}$
Corticotrophin$_{GB}$	*Acthar*$_{GB}$, used as alternative to **cortisone** and does not suppress adrenals
Cortisol$_{GB}$	see **hydrocortisone**$_{GB,US}$
Cortisone acetate$_{GB,US}$	a corticosteroid, causes adrenal suppression

Cotazym$_{GB,US}$	pancreatic supplement
Co-trimoxazole$_{GB}$	(*Bactrim*$_{GB,US}$, *Septrin*$_{GB}$), a mixture of **sulphamethoxazole** and **trimethoprim**
Cromolyn sodium$_{US}$	(*Intal*$_{US,GB}$), prophylactic agent in asthma
Cyanocobalamine$_{GB,US}$	vitamin B12 preparation now largely replaced by **hydroxocobalamin**
Cyclizine$_{GB,US}$	for nausea, vomiting, and vertigo
Cyclobarbitone$_{GB}$	barbiturate for severe intractable insomnia
Cyclopenthiazide$_{GB}$	(*Navidrex*$_{GB}$), diuretic
Cyclophosphamide$_{GB,US}$	(*Endoxana*$_{GB}$), (*Cytoxan*$_{US}$), cytotoxic agent, causes marrow depression
Cycloserine$_{GB,US}$	second line antituberculous agent
Cyklokapron$_{GB}$	see **tranexamic acid**$_{GB}$
Cysteamine$_{GB}$	antidote to **paracetamol** poisoning
Cytamen$_{GB}$	see **hydroxocobalamin**$_{GB}$
Cytarabine$_{GB,US}$	(*Cytosar*$_{US}$), cytotoxic agent, causes marrow depression
Cytosar$_{US}$	see **cytarabine**$_{GB,US}$
Cytoxan$_{US}$	see **cyclophosphamide**$_{GB,US}$

Dalacinc$_{GB}$	see **clindamycin**$_{GB,US}$
Dalmane$_{GB,US}$	see **flurazepam**$_{GB,US}$
Danthron$_{GB,US}$	(*Normatol*$_{GB}$), stimulant laxative
Dapsone$_{GB,US}$	a sulphone anti-leprotic drug, may cause oral erosions
Daraprim$_{GB,US}$	see **pyrimethamine**$_{GB,US}$
Daunorubicin$_{GB,US}$	cytotoxic agent, causes marrow depression
DDAVP$_{GB}$	a vasopressin analogue for use in diabetes insipidus
Debendox$_{GB}$	see **dicyclomine hydrochloride**$_{US,GB}$
Debrisoquine sulphate$_{GB}$	(*Declinax*$_{GB}$), adrenergic neurone blocking drug for moderate to severe hypertension; hypotensive effect of general anaesthetics potentiated
Decadron$_{GB,US}$	see **dexamethasone**$_{GB,US}$
Declinax$_{GB}$	see **debrisoquine sulphate**$_{GB}$
Declomycin$_{US}$	see **demeclocycline hydrochloride**$_{US,GB}$
Deglycyrrhizinized liquorice$_{GB}$	(*Caved-S*$_{GB}$), for treatment of peptic ulceration

Demeclocycline hydrochloride$_{US,GB}$	(*Ledermycin*$_{GB}$, *Declomycin*$_{US}$), antibiotic
De-Nol$_{GB}$	see **tripotassium dicitratobismuthate**$_{GB}$
Depixol$_{GB}$	see **flupenthixol**$_{GB}$
Depo-medrone$_{GB}$	*see* **methyl-prednisolone**$_{GB,US}$
Dermovate$_{GB}$	see **clobetasol proprionate**$_{GB}$
Deseril$_{GB}$	see **methylsergide**$_{GB,US}$
Desferrioxamine$_{GB}$	iron chelating agent used for iron overload
Deteclo$_{GB}$	see **tetracycline**$_{GB,US}$
Dexamethasone$_{US\ GB}$	(*Decadron*$_{US,GB}$), high-potency glucocorticoid with minimal mineralocorticoid action, may suppress adrenals
Dexamphetamine$_{GB}$	central nervous system stimulant; may give rise to drug-dependence
Dextromoramide$_{GB}$	(*Palfium*$_{GB}$), narcotic and analgesic for strong pain; may lead to dependence, avoid in patients on MAOIs
Dextropropoxyphene$_{GB}$	(*Depronal*$_{GB}$, *Distalgesic*$_{GB}$), narcotic analgesic for mild to moderate pain, potentiates **carbamazepine**
DF 118$_{GB}$	*see* **dihydrocodeine**$_{GB,US}$
Diamorphine$_{GB}$	(*Heroin*$_{GB}$), powerful narcotic analgesic likely to lead to dependence, not to be given to patients taking MAOIs
Diamox$_{GB,US}$	see **acetazolamide**$_{GB,US}$
Diazepam$_{GB,US}$	(*Valium*$_{GB,US}$), hypnotic with a wide range of actions including anxiolytic pre-medication and anti-epileptic, effect prolonged by **cimetidine**
Diazoxide$_{GB,US}$	(*Eudemine*$_{GB}$), vasodilator hypotensive; may cause hyperglycaemia
Dibenyline$_{GB}$	see **phenoxybenzamine**$_{US,GB}$
Dibotin$_{GB}$	see **phenformin**
Dichloralphenazone$_{GB,US}$	(*Welldorm*$_{GB,US}$), mild sedative
Diclofenac$_{GB}$	(*Voltarol*$_{GB}$), non-steroidal anti-inflammatory agent
Diconal$_{GB}$	see **dipipanone**$_{GB}$
Dicoumarol$_{GB,US}$	(*Warfarin*$_{GB}$), anticoagulant, (*Dicumarol*$_{US}$), potentiated by **aspirin, mefenamic acid,** and **metronidazole**
Dicumarol$_{US}$	anticoagulant

Dicyclomine$_{US,GB}$ (*Merbentyl*$_{GB}$), antispasmodic, may cause dry mouth

Diethylpropion$_{GB,US}$ (*Apisate*$_{GB}$, *Tenuate*$_{GB,US}$), centrally acting appetite-suppressant

Diflunisal$_{GB}$ (*Dolobid*$_{GB}$), long-acting analgesic for mild to moderate pain

Digoxin$_{GB,US}$ cardiac glycoside used in atrial dysrhythmias

Dihydrocodeine$_{GB,US}$ (*DF 118*), analgesic

Dilantin$_{US}$ see **phenytoin**$_{GB,US}$

Dimelor$_{GB}$ see **acetohexamide**$_{GB,US}$

Dimenhydrinate$_{GB,US}$ (*Dramamine*$_{GB,US}$), antihistamine

Dindevan$_{GB}$ see **phenindione**$_{GB}$

Diphenhydramine$_{US,GB}$ (*Benadryl*$_{US,GB}$), antihistamine

Diphenoxylate$_{GB,US}$ (*Lomotil*$_{GB}$), anti-diarrhoeal agent, may cause a dry mouth

Dipipanone$_{GB}$ (*Diconal*$_{GB}$), narcotic analgesic, not to be given to patients on MAOIs

Dipyridamole$_{GB,US}$ (*Persantin*$_{GB,US}$) anti-platelet agent

Disipal$_{US,GB}$ see **orphenadrine**$_{GB,US}$

Disopyramide$_{US,GB}$ (*Rythmodan*$_{GB}$), used in ventricular arrhythmias, may cause a dry mouth

Distalgesic$_{GB}$ see **dextropropoxyphane**$_{GB}$

Disulfiram$_{GB,US}$ (*Antabuse*$_{GB,US}$), used in treatment of alcoholism

Dixarit$_{GB}$ see **clonidine**$_{US,GB}$

Dolobid$_{GB}$ see **diflunisal**$_{GB}$

Dopamine$_{GB,US}$ (*Intropin*$_{US}$), sympathomimetic agent used in cardiogenic shock

Dopram$_{GB,US}$ see **doxapram**$_{GB,US}$

Dorbanex$_{GB}$ see **danthron**$_{GB,US}$

Doriden$_{US GB}$ see **glutethimide**$_{US,GB}$

Dothiepin$_{GB}$ (*Prothiaden*$_{GB}$), tricyclic antidepressant, may cause a dry mouth, use LAs without **adrenaline**

Doxapram$_{GB,US}$ (*Dopram*$_{GB,US}$), respiratory stimulant

Doxorubicin hydrochloride$_{GB,US}$ cytotoxic agent

Dramamine$_{US,GB}$ see **dimenhydrinate**$_{GB,US}$

Droperidol$_{GB,US}$ for tranquillization and control of psychoses

Duogastrone$_{\text{GB}}$	see **carbonoxolone sodium**$_{\text{GB}}$
Duphaston$_{\text{GB}}$	see **dydrogesterone**$_{\text{GB}}$
Durabolin$_{\text{GB,US}}$	see **nandrolone**$_{\text{GB,US}}$
Dyazide$_{\text{GB,US}}$	see **triamterene**$_{\text{GB,US}}$
Dydrogesterone$_{\text{GB}}$	(*Duphaston*$_{\text{GB}}$), progestogen
Dytac$_{\text{GB}}$	see **triamterene**$_{\text{GB,US}}$
Dytide$_{\text{GB}}$	see **triamterene + benzthiazide**$_{\text{GB,US}}$
Edecrin$_{\text{GB,US}}$	see **ethacrinic acid**$_{\text{GB,US}}$
Edrophonium$_{\text{GB,US}}$	(*Tensilon*$_{\text{GB,US}}$), used for the diagnosis of myasthenia
Efcortelan$_{\text{GB}}$	**hydrocortisone cream**
Eltroxin$_{\text{GB}}$	see **thyroxin**$_{\text{GB,US}}$
Emepronium bromide$_{\text{GB}}$	(*Cetiprin*$_{\text{GB}}$), for urinary incontinence; oral and oesophageal ulceration have been described as complications
Emeside$_{\text{GB}}$	see **ethosuximide**$_{\text{GB,US}}$
Emetine$_{\text{GB}}$	amoebicide
Endoxana$_{\text{GB}}$	see **cyclophosphamide**$_{\text{GB,US}}$
Epanutin$_{\text{GB}}$	see **phenytoin**$_{\text{GB,US}}$
Epilim$_{\text{GB}}$	see **sodium valproate**$_{\text{GB}}$
Epsikapron$_{\text{GB}}$	see **aminocaproic acid**$_{\text{GB,US}}$
Equagesic$_{\text{GB,US}}$	compound analgesic
Equanil$_{\text{GB,US}}$	see **meprobamate**$_{\text{GB,US}}$
Eraldin$_{\text{GB}}$	see **practolol**$_{\text{GB}}$
Ergotamine tartrate$_{\text{GB,US}}$	constricts cranial arteries; used in migraine and vascular headaches; should never be used prophylactically
Erythrocin$_{\text{GB,US}}$	see **erythromycin**$_{\text{GB,US}}$
Erythromycin$_{\text{GB,US}}$	antibiotic with similar spectrum to **penicillin** (*Erythrocin*$_{\text{GB,US}}$, *Ilosone*$_{\text{GB,US}}$)
Esbatal$_{\text{GB}}$	see **bethanidine**$_{\text{GB}}$
Ethacrynic acid$_{\text{GB,US}}$	(*Edecrin*$_{\text{US,GB}}$), loop diuretic, strong and of similar action to **frusemide**
Ethambutol$_{\text{GB,US}}$	(*Mynah*$_{\text{GB}}$), antituberculous drug; should be avoided in the very young and the elderly
Ethionamide$_{\text{GB,US}}$	antituberculous drug used where resistance to first-line drugs occurs
Ethosuximide$_{\text{GB,US}}$	(*Zarontin*$_{\text{GB,US}}$, *Emeside*$_{\text{GB}}$), used in treatment of petit mal

Fansidar$_{GB}$	see **pyrimethamine**$_{GB,US}$ + **sulfadoxine**$_{GB}$
Fefol$_{GB}$	**iron + folate** preparation
Feldene$_{GB}$	see **piroxicam**$_{GB}$
Fenfluramine$_{GB,US}$	(*Ponderax*$_{GB}$, *Pondimin*$_{US}$), appetite-suppressant, may be a hazard for general anaesthetics
Fenoprofen$_{GB,US}$	(*Progesic*$_{GB}$), non-steroidal anti-inflammatory analgesic, absorption impaired by **aspirin**
Fentazin$_{GB}$	see **perphenazine**$_{GB,US}$
Flagyl$_{GB,US}$	see **metranidazole**$_{GB,US}$
Flavoxate$_{GB,US}$	(*Urispas*$_{GB,US}$), for urinary frequency and dysuria
Floxapen$_{GB}$	see **flucloxacillin**$_{GB}$
Flucloxacillin$_{GB}$	penicillinase-resistant **penicillin** for use in penicillin-resistant **Staphylococcus aureus** infections
Fludrocortisone$_{GB,US}$	salt-retaining steroid used for replacement therapy in mineralocorticoid deficiency, may suppress adrenals
Flufenamic acid$_{GB}$	(*Meralen*$_{GB}$) non-steroidal anti-inflammatory analgesic
Fluorouracil$_{GB,US}$	antimetabolite used for cancer therapy, may cause marrow depression
Flupenthixol$_{GB}$	(*Depixol*$_{GB}$), used for psychoses and related disorders
Fluphenazine$_{GB,US}$	(*Modecate*$_{GB}$), used for psychoses and related disorders
Flurazepam$_{GB,US}$	(*Dalmane*$_{GB,US}$), hypnotic and anxiolytic
Flurbiprofen$_{GB}$	(*Froben*$_{GB}$), anti-inflammatory analgesic
Fortagesic$_{GB}$	compound analgesic
Fortral$_{GB}$	see **pentazocine**$_{GB,US}$
Fosfestrol$_{GB}$	(*Honvan*$_{GB}$), converted to **stilboestrol**; used in malignant disease, e.g. prostatic carcinoma
Framycetin$_{GB}$	(*Soframycin*$_{GB}$), almost identical to **neomycin** in its actions and uses
Franol$_{GB}$	compound preparation **ephedrine**$_{GB,US}$, **theophylline**$_{GB,US}$, **phenobarbitone**$_{GB,US}$
Froben$_{GB}$	see **flurbiprofen**$_{GB}$

Frusemide$_{\text{GB}}$	(*Lasix*$_{\text{GB,US}}$), powerful loop diuretic, oral erosions have been reported
Fucidin$_{\text{GB}}$	see **sodium fusidate**$_{\text{GB}}$
Fulcin$_{\text{GB}}$	see **griseofulvin**$_{\text{GB,US}}$
Fulvicin$_{\text{US}}$	see **griseofulvin**$_{\text{GB,US}}$
Fungilin$_{\text{GB}}$	see **amphotericin**$_{\text{GB,US}}$
Fungizone$_{\text{US,GB}}$	see **amphotericin**$_{\text{GB,US}}$
Furadantin$_{\text{GB,US}}$	see **nitrofurantoin**$_{\text{GB,US}}$
Furosemide$_{\text{US}}$	(*Lasix*), loop diuretic, oral erosions have been reported
Fybogel$_{\text{GB}}$	see **ispaghula husk**$_{\text{GB}}$
Gamma benzene hexachloride$_{\text{GB,US}}$	(*Lorexane*$_{\text{GB}}$), for treatment of lice and scabies
Garamycin$_{\text{GB,US}}$	see **gentamicin**$_{\text{GB,US}}$
Gastrocote$_{\text{GB}}$	compound antacid
Gaviscon$_{\text{GB,US}}$	compound antacid
Gelusil$_{\text{GB,US}}$	compound antacid
Gentamicin$_{\text{GB,US}}$	(*Genticin*$_{\text{GB}}$, *Garamycin*$_{\text{GB,US}}$), most important aminoglycoside antibiotic, broad spectrum; may cause renal and hepatic damage if blood levels become too high
Genticin$_{\text{GB}}$	see **gentamicin**$_{\text{GB,US}}$
Glibenclamide$_{\text{GB}}$	(*Daonil*$_{\text{GB}}$, *Euglucon*$_{\text{GB}}$), oral hypoglycaemic agent, potentiated by **aspirin**
Glutethimide$_{\text{GB,US}}$	(*Doriden*$_{\text{GB,US}}$), sedative
Glyceryl trinitrate$_{\text{GB,US}}$	vasodilator commonly used in angina pectoris
Griseofulvin$_{\text{GB,US}}$	(*Fulcin*$_{\text{GB}}$, *Grisovin*$_{\text{GB}}$), anti-fungal agent used for severe dermatophyte infections, may cause loss of taste
Grisovin$_{\text{GB}}$	see **griseofulvin**$_{\text{GB,US}}$
Guanethidine$_{\text{GB,US}}$	(*Ismelin*$_{\text{GB,US}}$), adrenergic neurone-blocking agent used for hypertension, hypotensive effect of general anaesthetics potentiated, may cause parotid gland discomfort

Halcion$_{GB}$ see **triazolam**$_{GB}$

Haloperidol$_{GB,US}$ (*Serenace*$_{GB}$), used in acute and chronic schizophrenia and related disorders

Harmogen$_{GB}$ see **piperazine oestrone sulphate**$_{GB,US}$

Hashish$_{GB}$ see **marihuana**$_{GB}$

Heminevrin$_{GB}$ see **chlormethiazole**$_{GB}$

Heparin$_{GB,US}$ anticoagulant

Heroin$_{GB}$ see **diamorphine**$_{GB}$

Herpid$_{GB}$ see **idoxuridine**$_{GB}$, *Herpid* is a colourless solution containing 5 per cent **idoxuridine** in 100 per cent **dimethyl sulphoxide**

Hexochlorophane$_{GB,US}$ (*Zalpon cidal soap*$_{GB}$), active against Gram-positive organisms

Hexopal$_{GB}$ see **inositol nicotinate**$_{GB,US}$

Hiprex$_{GB}$ see **hexamine**$_{GB}$

Homatropine$_{GB,US}$ (mydriatic)

Honvan$_{GB}$ see **fosfestrol**$_{GB}$

Hydergine$_{GB,US}$ see **co-dergocrine mesylate**$_{GB,US}$

Hydralazine$_{GB,US}$ (*Apresoline*$_{GB,US}$), hypotensive agent active on the central nervous system; may give rise to a rheumatoid arthritis-like syndrome or sometimes a picture resembling disseminated lupus erythematosus

Hydrochlorothiazide$_{GB,US}$ (*Hydrosaluric*$_{GB}$), also contained in *Moduretic, Cobetaloc, Diazide,* and *Hydromet*; a diuretic used for mild hypertension

Hydrocortisone$_{GB,US}$ (*Cortisol*$_{GB}$), the principal naturally occurring steroid. The soluble salt (**hydrocortisone sodium succinate**) can be given intravenously for rapid effect in an emergency. A suspension of the insoluble **hydrocortisone acetate** can be given intramuscularly for prolonged effect, and also intra-articularly

Hydroflumethiazide$_{GB,US}$ contained in *Rautrax*$_{GB}$ (**Rauwolfia serpentina** plus **hydroflumethiazide**) and *Aldactide*$_{GB}$ (**spironolactone** plus **hydroflumethiazide**), a thiazide diuretic

Hydromet$_{GB}$ see **methyldopa**$_{GB,US}$

Hydrosaluric$_{GB}$	see **hydrochlorothiazide**$_{GB,US}$
Hydrotalcite$_{GB}$	(*Altacite*$_{GB}$), antacid
Hydroxocobalamin$_{GB}$	(vitamin B12, *Neo-Cytamen*$_{GB}$), given parenterally as maintenance therapy, usually 1000 μg monthly
Hydroxychloroquine sulphate$_{GB,US}$	(*Plaquenil*$_{GB,US}$), used in treatment of malaria, rheumatoid arthritis, and lupus erythematosus; can cause oral erosions
Hydroxycholecalciferol$_{GB}$	vitamin D
Hydroxyurea$_{GB,US}$	an orally active cytotoxic agent; probably acting by interfering with synthesis of deoxyribonucleic acid, may cause marrow depression
Hygroton$_{GB,US}$	see **chlorthalidone**$_{GB,US}$
Hyoscine$_{GB,US}$	(*Scopolamine*$_{GB,US}$), chemically related to **atropine**; anticholinergic, used for its mydriatic and cycloplegic properties; may cause confusion
Hypovase$_{GB}$	see **prazosin**$_{GB,US}$
Ibuprofen$_{GB,US}$	(*Brufen*$_{GB}$), non-steroidal anti-inflammatory agent
Idoxuridine$_{GB}$	(*Herpid*$_{GB}$), antiviral agent
Ilosone$_{GB,US}$	see **erythromycin**$_{GB,US}$
Imipramine$_{GB,US}$	tricyclic antidepressant, use LAs without **adrenaline**; may cause dryness of the mouth
Imodium$_{GB,US}$	see **loperamide**$_{GB,US}$
Imuran$_{GB,US}$	see **azathioprine**$_{GB,US}$
Indapamide$_{GB}$	(*Natrilix*$_{GB}$), thiazide-like agent used for mild hypertension
Inapasade$_{GB}$	**aminosalicylic acid** + **isoniazid**$_{GB,US}$
Inderal$_{GB,US}$	see **propanolol**$_{GB,US}$
Indocid$_{GB}$	see **indomethacin**$_{GB,US}$
Indocin$_{US}$	see **indomethacin**$_{GB,US}$
Indomethacin$_{GB,US}$	(*Indocid*$_{GB}$) (*Indocin*$_{US}$) non-steroidal anti-inflammatory agent, oral ulceration has been reported
Influvac$_{GB}$	influenza vaccine
Inositol$_{GB}$	one of the vitamin B group

Insulin$_{GB,US}$ treatment of diabetes mellitus, salivary gland enlargement has been reported

Intal$_{GB,US}$ see **sodium chromoglycate**$_{GB,US}$

Intropin$_{US}$ see **dopamine**$_{GB,US}$

Ipecacuanha$_{GB,US}$ expectorant

Ipratropium bromide$_{GB}$ (*Atrovent*$_{GB}$), anticholinergic drug used for bronchospasm in chronic bronchitis

Iproniazid$_{GB}$ (*Marsilid*$_{GB}$), MAOI used for depressive illness; **amphetamine, ephedrine,** and narcotic analgesics to be avoided

Ismelin$_{GB,US}$ see **guanethidine**$_{GB,US}$

Isocarboxazid$_{GB,US}$ (*Marplan*$_{GB,US}$), MAOI used for depressive illness; **amphetamine, ephedrine,** and narcotic analgesics to be avoided

Isogel$_{GB}$ see **ispaghula husk**$_{GB}$

Isoniazid$_{GB,US}$ anti-tuberculous drug; interferes with the metabolism of vitamin B6, may cause stomatitis, angular cheilitis, and oral ulceration

Isoprenaline$_{GB}$ (*Saventrine*$_{GB}$), sympathomimetic agent used in heart block and bronchospasm, can cause parotid swelling and oral ulceration, use LAs without **adrenaline** and avoid **halothane**

Isordil$_{GB,US}$ see **isosorbide dinitrate**$_{GB,US}$

Isosorbide dinitrate$_{GB,US}$ (*Isordil*$_{GB,US}$), long-acting nitrate used for angina

Ispaghula husk$_{GB}$ (*Isogel*$_{GB}$), adsorbent agent used for diarrhoea

Jectofer$_{GB}$ injectable iron

Juvel$_{GB}$ multivitamin

Kanamycin$_{GB,US}$ antibiotic for serious Gram-negative infections resistant to **gentamicin**; care needed with renal impairment

Kaolin$_{GB,US}$ adsorbent anti-diarrhoeal agent

Kaomycin$_{GB}$ **kaolin**$_{GB,US}$ + **neomycin**$_{GB,US}$

Kaopectate$_{GB,US}$ see **kaolin**$_{GB,US}$

Keflex$_{GB,US}$ see **cephalexin**$_{GB,US}$

Keflin$_{GB,US}$ — see **cephalothin**$_{GB,US}$
Kemicetine$_{GB}$ — see **chloramphenicol**$_{GB,US}$
Kenalog in orobase$_{US}$ — see **triamcinolone paste**$_{GB,US}$
Ketoprofen$_{GB}$ — (*Alrheumat*$_{GB}$, *Orudis*$_{GB}$), anti-inflammatory agent similar to **ibuprofen**
Keto tifen$_{GB}$ — (*Zaditen*$_{GB}$), for prophylaxis in asthma, may cause a dry mouth
Kinidin$_{GB}$ — see **quinidine**$_{GB,US}$
Kloref$_{GB}$ — see **potassium chloride**$_{GB,US}$

Labetalol$_{GB}$ — (*Trandate*$_{GB}$), alpha- and beta-adrenoceptor blocker for hypertension, potentiates hypotensive effect of general anaesthetics
Lactulose$_{GB,US}$ — (*Duphulac*$_{GB}$), osmotic laxative used for constipation and in hepatic encephalopathy
Lanoxin$_{GB,US}$ — see **digoxin**$_{GB,US}$
Largactil$_{GB}$ — see **chlorpromazine**$_{GB,US}$
Lasikal$_{GB}$ — **frusemide**$_{GB}$ + **potassium**$_{GB,US}$
Lasix$_{GB,US}$ — see **frusemide**$_{GB}$; see **furosemide**$_{US}$
Ledercort$_{GB}$ — see **triamcinolone**$_{GB,US}$
Ledermycin$_{GB}$ — see **demeclocycline**$_{GB,US}$
Lentizol$_{GB}$ — see **amitriptyline**$_{GB,US}$
Leukeran$_{GB,US}$ — see **chlorambucil**$_{GB,US}$
Levodopa$_{GB,US}$ — (*Madopar*$_{GB}$, *Sinemet*$_{GB,US}$), dopaminergic drug used in Parkinsonism; avoid use of **halothane**
Libraxin$_{GB}$ — **chlordiazepoxide**$_{GB,US}$ + **clidinium bromide**$_{GB,US}$
Librium$_{GB,US}$ — see **chlordiazepoxide**$_{GB,US}$
Limbritol$_{GB,US}$ — see **amitriptyline**$_{GB,US}$ + **chlordiazepoxide**$_{GB,US}$
Lincocin$_{GB,US}$ — see **lincomycin**
Lincomycin$_{GB,US}$ — (*Lincocin*$_{GB,US}$), active against Gram-positive cocci, but use limited by serious side-effects, especially pseudomembranous colitis
Lithium carbonate$_{GB,US}$ — (*Priadel*$_{GB}$), prevention of mania and manic depressive illness

Lomotil$_{\text{GB,US}}$	see **diphenoxylate**$_{\text{GB,US}}$
Lomustine$_{\text{GB,US}}$	(*CCNU*$_{\text{GB,US}}$), cytotoxic agent, causes marrow depression
Loperamide$_{\text{GB,US}}$	(*Imodium*$_{\text{GB,US}}$), anti-diarrhoeal agent
Lopresor$_{\text{GB,US}}$	see **metoprolol**$_{\text{GB,US}}$
Lopurin$_{\text{US}}$	see **allopurinol**$_{\text{GB,US}}$
Lorazepam$_{\text{GB,US}}$	(*Ativan*$_{\text{GB,US}}$), anxiolytic agent
Loridine$_{\text{US}}$	see **cephaloridine**$_{\text{GB,US}}$
Luminal$_{\text{GB,US}}$	see **phenobarbitone**$_{\text{GB,US}}$
Lysergic acid$_{\text{GB}}$	LSD. Class A controlled drug
Lysine vasopressin$_{\text{GB,US}}$	*Lypressin*$_{\text{GB,US}}$ posterior pituitary hormone for diabetes insipidus
Maalox$_{\text{GB,US}}$	compound antacid
Madopar$_{\text{GB}}$	**Levodopa**$_{\text{GB,US}}$ + **benserazide**$_{\text{GB}}$
Magnapen$_{\text{GB}}$	**ampicillin**$_{\text{GB,US}}$ + **flucloxacillin**$_{\text{GB}}$
Magnesium trisilicate$_{\text{GB,US}}$	antacid
Malathion$_{\text{GB}}$	(*Derbac*$_{\text{GB}}$), used for lice and scabies infection
Mandelamine$_{\text{GB,US}}$	see **hexamine mandelate**$_{\text{GB,US}}$
Marcain$_{\text{GB,US}}$	see **bupivacaine**$_{\text{GB,US}}$
Marevan$_{\text{GB}}$	see **warfarin**$_{\text{GB,US}}$
Marplan$_{\text{GB,US}}$	see **isocarboxazid**$_{\text{GB,US}}$
Marsalid$_{\text{GB}}$	see **iproniazid**$_{\text{GB}}$
Matulane$_{\text{US}}$	see **procarbazine**$_{\text{GB,US}}$
Maxolon$_{\text{GB}}$	see **metoclopramide**$_{\text{GB,US}}$
Mebendazole$_{\text{GB,US}}$	(*Vermox*$_{\text{GB,US}}$), for treatment of threadworm, roundworm, and hookworm
Mebeverine$_{\text{GB}}$	(*Colofac*$_{\text{GB}}$), anti-spasmodic for colonic spasm
Mefenamic acid$_{\text{GB,US}}$	(*Ponstan*$_{\text{GB,US}}$), analgesic for mild to moderate pain, potentiates action of **warfarin**
Mefruside$_{\text{GB}}$	diuretic
Melleril$_{\text{GB,US}}$	see **thioridazine**$_{\text{GB,US}}$
Melphalan$_{\text{GB,US}}$	(*Alkeran*$_{\text{GB,US}}$), cytotoxic agent for myelomatosis, causes marrow depression
Menadiol sodium phosphate$_{\text{GB,US}}$	(*Synkavit*$_{\text{GB,US}}$, *Synkayvite*$_{\text{US}}$) vitamin K, water soluble by mouth or injection
Mepacrine$_{\text{GB}}$	used for tapeworm infestation, known to cause oral erosions

Meprobamate$_{GB,US}$ — (*Equanil*$_{GB,US}$), anxiolytic for mild anxiety

Mepyramine$_{GB}$ — antihistamine for nasal allergy and urticaria

Meralen$_{GB}$ — see **flufenamic acid**$_{GB}$

Merbentyl$_{GB}$ — see **dicyclomine**$_{GB,US}$

Mercaptopurine$_{GB,US}$ — antimetabolite used in acute leukaemia, suppresses bone marrow

Merital$_{GB}$ — see **nomifensine**$_{GB}$

Mersalyl$_{GB}$ — mercurial diuretic

Mestinon$_{GB,US}$ — see **pyridostigmine**$_{GB,US}$

Mestranol$_{GB,US}$ — contraceptive, occasionally causes light pigmentation in the mouth

Metformin$_{GB}$ — (*Glucophage*$_{GB}$), biguanide oral hypoglycaemic agent

Methadone$_{GB,US}$ — (*Physeptone*$_{GB}$), strong analgesic used in oral treatment of chronic pain in terminal disease, to be avoided in patients on MAOIs

Methicillin$_{GB,US}$ — parenteral **penicillin** for infections due to penicillinase-producing staphylococci

Methimazole$_{US}$ — (*tapazole*$_{US}$), treatment of hyperthyroidism, may cause loss of taste

Methotrexate$_{GB,US}$ — antimetabolite, depresses bone marrow, toxicity increased by aspirin

Methyl cellulose$_{GB,US}$ — bulk-forming laxative

Methyldopa$_{GB,US}$ — (*Aldomet*$_{GB,US}$), hypotensive agent, can cause oral erosions and parotid discomfort

Methyl prednisolone$_{GB,US}$ — glucocorticoid, suppresses adrenals

Methysergide$_{GB,US}$ — (*Deseril*$_{GB}$, *Sansent*$_{US}$), anti-serotonergic agent used in migraine and neuralgia

Metoclopramide$_{GB,US}$ — (*Maxolon*$_{GB}$), used for digestive disorders, speeds gastric emptying, used for nausea

Metoprolol$_{GB,US}$ — (*Betaloc*$_{GB}$, *Lopresor*$_{GB,US}$), beta-blocker used for hypertension and angina, hypotensive effect of general anaesthetics potentiated

Metronidazole$_{GB,US}$ — (*Flagyl*$_{GB,US}$), antimicrobial agent highly active against anaerobic bacteria and protozoa, potentiates action of **warfarin**

Mexiletine$_{GB}$ — dysrhythmic agent used for ventricular arrhythmias

Mianserine$_{GB}$	tricyclic antidepressant, use LAs without **adrenaline**
Midrin$_{US}$	see **dichloralphenazone**$_{GB,US}$
Migraleve$_{GB}$	combination anti-migraine preparation
Migravess$_{GB}$	combination anti-migraine preparation
Migril$_{GB}$	see **ergotamine tartrate**$_{GB,US}$, treatment for migraine
Minipress$_{US}$	see **prazosin**$_{GB,US}$
Mithramycin$_{GB,US}$	cytotoxic antibiotic useful for hypercalcaemia associated with malignancy, causes marked marrow depression
Mitomycin$_{GB,US}$	cytotoxic antibiotic used for gastrointestinal tumours, causes marrow depression
Modecate$_{GB}$	see **fluphenazine**$_{GB,US}$
Moduretic$_{GB}$	**amiloride**$_{GB}$ + **hydrochlorothiazide**$_{GB,US}$
Mogadon$_{GB}$	see **nitrazepam**$_{GB}$
Monotard	*see* **insulin**$_{GB,US}$
Morphine$_{GB,US}$	narcotic analgesic, not to be used in patients on MAOIs
Motipress$_{GB}$	**fluphenazine**$_{GB,US}$ + **nortriptyline**$_{GB,US}$
Motival$_{GB}$	**fluphenazine**$_{GB,US}$ + **nortriptyline**$_{GB,US}$
MST 1$_{GB}$	oral preparation of **morphine sulphate**, not to be used on patients on MAOIs
Mucaine$_{GB}$	antacid
Mustine$_{GB}$	alkylating drug particularly valuable in the treatment of Hodgkin's, depresses bone marrow
Mycardol$_{GB}$	see **pentaerythritol tetranitrate**$_{GB,US}$
Mycelex$_{US}$	see **clotrimazole**$_{GB,US}$
Mycostatin$_{US}$	see **nystatin**$_{US,GB}$
Myleran$_{GB,US}$	see **busulphan**$_{GB,US}$
Myocrisin$_{GB,US}$	see **sodium aurothiomalate**$_{GB,US}$
Mysoline$_{GB,US}$	see **primidone**$_{GB,US}$
Mysteclin$_{GB,US}$	**tetracycline** + **amphotericin B**$_{GB,US}$

Nacton$_{GB}$	see **poldine methylsulphate**$_{GB}$
Nadolol$_{GB,US}$	(*Corgard*$_{GB,US}$), beta-blocker for angina and hypertension, hypotensive effect of general anaesthetics potentiated

Nalcrom$_{GB}$	see **sodium cromoglycate**$_{GB}$
Nalidixic acid$_{GB,US}$	(*Negram*$_{GB,US}$), urinary antibiotic
Naloxone$_{GB,US}$	(*Narcan*$_{GB,US}$) antidote to morphine-like drugs
Nandrolone$_{GB,US}$	(*Durabolin*$_{GB,US}$), anabolic steroid
Naprosyn$_{GB,US}$	see **naproxen**$_{GB,US}$
Naproxen$_{GB,US}$	(*Naprosyn*$_{GB,US}$), anti-inflammatory analgesic
Narcan$_{GB,US}$	see **naloxone**$_{GB,US}$
Nardil$_{GB,US}$	see **phenelzine**$_{GB,US}$
Natrilix$_{GB}$	see **indapamide**$_{GB}$
Natulan$_{GB}$	see **procarbazine**$_{GB,US}$
Navidrex$_{GB}$	see **cyclopenthiazide**$_{GB}$
Nefopam$_{GB}$	(*Acupan*$_{GB}$), powerful non-narcotic analgesic
Negram$_{GB,US}$	see **nalidixic acid**$_{GB,US}$
Nembutal$_{GB,US}$	see **pentobarbitone**$_{GB,US}$
Neo-cytamen$_{GB}$	see **hydroxocobalamin**$_{GB}$
Neo-mercazole$_{GB}$	see **carbimazole**$_{GB}$
Neomycin$_{GB,US}$	non-parenteral aminoglycoside antibiotic
Neo-naclex$_{GB}$	see **bendrofluazide**$_{GB}$
Neostigmine$_{GB,US}$	anticholinesterase for diagnosis and treatment of myasthenia gravis
Nepenthe$_{GB}$	see **morphine**$_{GB,US}$
Neutradonna$_{GB}$	see **belladonna**$_{GB,US}$
Nifedipine$_{GB}$	(*Adalat*$_{GB}$), for angina
Nikethamide$_{GB,US}$	respiratory stimulant
Nitrates$_{GB,US}$	for angina
Nitrazepam$_{GB}$	(*Mogadon*$_{GB}$), sedative
Nitrofurantoin$_{GB,US}$	(*Furadantin*$_{GB,US}$), urinary antibiotic
Nomifensine$_{GB}$	(*Merital*$_{GB}$), for depressive illness associated with anxiety
Noradrenaline$_{GB}$	
Norethandrolone$_{GB}$	(*Nilevar*$_{GB}$), anabolic steroid
Norethisterone$_{GB}$	sex hormone, contraceptive, and used in uterine dysfunction, occasionally causes light pigmentation in the mouth
Norgesic$_{GB,US}$	compound analgesic, avoid in patients with glaucoma
Normacol$_{GB}$	see **sterculia**$_{GB}$
Nortriptyline$_{GB,US}$	tricyclic antidepressant, use LAs without **adrenaline**; may cause dryness of the mouth

Nulacin$_{GB}$	antacid
Nutrizym$_{GB}$	pancreatic enzyme
Nystatin$_{GB,US}$	(*Mycostatin*$_{US}$), anti-fungal agent for candidiasis
Omnopon$_{GB}$	see **papaveretum**$_{GB}$
Oncovin$_{GB,US}$	see **vincristine**$_{GB,US}$
Optimax$_{GB}$	see **tryptophan**$_{GB}$
Orciprenaline$_{GB}$	(*Alupent*$_{GB}$), adrenoceptor stimulant for bronchospasm
Orphenadrine$_{GB,US}$	(*Disipal*$_{GB,US}$), for Parkinsonism, anticholinergic
Orudis$_{GB}$	see **ketoprofen**$_{GB}$
Ospolot$_{GB}$	see **sulthiame**$_{GB}$
Ouabain$_{GB}$	cardiac glycoside for supraventricular dysrhythmias and heart failure
Oxazepam$_{GB,US}$	short-acting anxiolytic
Oxprenolol$_{GB}$	(*Trasicor*$_{GB}$), beta-blocker, hypotensive effect of general anaesthetics potentiated
Oxymetazoline$_{GB,US}$	(*Afrazine*$_{GB}$, *Ilidine*$_{GB}$, *Alfrin*$_{US}$), nasal drop decongestant; avoid in patients on MAOIs
Oxymetholone$_{GB,US}$	(*Anapolon*$_{GB}$), anabolic steroid
Oxyphenbutazone$_{GB,US}$	(*Tanderil*$_{GB}$, *Tandearil*$_{US}$), non-steroidal anti-inflammatory analgesic, may cause oral ulceration and enlargement of salivary glands
Oxytetracycline$_{GB,US}$	tetracycline antibiotic
Oxytocin$_{GB,US}$	(*Pitocin*$_{GB,US}$, *Syntocinon*$_{GB,US}$), myometrial stimulant
Palfium$_{GB}$	see **dextromoramide**$_{GB}$
Paludrine$_{GB}$	see **proguanil**$_{GB}$
Panadol$_{GB}$	see **paracetamol**$_{GB}$
Pancrex$_{GB}$	**pancreatic enzyme**
Papaveretum$_{GB}$	(*Omnopon*$_{GB}$), narcotic analgesic, avoid in patients on MAOIs
Paracetamol$_{GB}$	(*Panadol*$_{GB}$), mild analgesic, overdosage may lead to severe liver damage, potentiated by **metoclopramide**
Paraldehyde$_{GB,US}$	occasionally used for status epilepticus

Paramax$_{GB}$	combination preparation for migraine
Parnate$_{GB,US}$	see **tranylcypromine**$_{GB,US}$
Parstelin$_{GB}$	**tranylcypromine**$_{GB,US}$ + **trifluoperazine**$_{GB,US}$
Pavulon$_{GB,US}$	see **pancuronium**$_{GB,US}$
Penbritin$_{GB}$	see **ampicillin**$_{GB,US}$
Penicillamine$_{GB,US}$	used in severe active rheumatoid arthritis, Wilson's disease and cystinuria, may cause loss of taste and oral manifestations of pemphigus
Penicillin$_{GB,US}$	bactericidal antibiotic
Pentaerythritol tetranitrate$_{GB,US}$	(*Mycardol*$_{GB}$, *Peritrate*$_{GB,US}$), prophylaxis of angina
Pentazocine$_{GB,US}$	(*Fortral*$_{GB}$, *Talwin*$_{US}$), analgesic for moderate to severe pain
Pentobarbitone	(*Nembutal*$_{GB,US}$), sedative
Perhexiline maleate$_{GB}$	(*Pexid*$_{GB}$), for angina
Peritrate$_{GB,US}$	see **pentaerythritol tetranitrate**$_{GB,US}$
Perphenazine$_{GB,US}$	(*Fentazin*$_{GB}$), anti-nausea, also schizophrenia and related psychoses
Persantin$_{GB,US}$	see **dipyridamole**$_{GB,US}$
Pethidine$_{GB}$	narcotic analgesic, avoid in patients on MAOIs
Pexid$_{GB}$	see **perhexiline maleate**$_{GB}$
Phenacetin$_{GB,US}$	analgesic; prolonged use leads to serious renal damage
Phenelzine$_{GB,US}$	(*Nardil*$_{US,GB}$), MAOI for depressive illness, **amphetamine, ephedrine,** and narcotic analgesics to be avoided
Phenergan$_{GB,US}$	see **promethazine**$_{GB,US}$
Phenformin$_{GB}$	(*Dibotin*$_{GB}$), biguanide hypoglycaemic agent for diabetes mellitus
Pheniramine maleate$_{GB,US}$	(*Daneral*$_{GB}$), antihistamine
Phenobarbitone$_{GB,US}$	barbiturate little used now as a sedative, but occasionally used in epilepsy
Phenoperidine$_{GB}$	used for analgesia in operations
Phenoxybenzamine$_{GB,US}$	(*Dibenyline*$_{GB}$, *Dibenzyline*$_{US}$), alpha-adrenergic blocker used to control hypertension in phaeochromocytomas
Phensedyl$_{GB}$	cough linctus

Phentolamine$_{GB,US}$	(*Regitine*$_{US}$, *Rogitine*$_{GB}$), alpha-adrenergic blocker; indications as for **phenoxybenzamine**
Phenylbutazone$_{GB,US}$	(*Butazolidin*$_{GB,US}$) non-steroidal anti-inflammatory analgesic; may cause serious gastrointestinal haemorrhage, and oral ulceration and parotid enlargement
Phenylephrine$_{GB,US}$	sympathomimetic agent for hypotension and used in eye drops as a mydriatic
Phenytoin$_{GB,US}$	(*Epanutin*$_{GB}$) *Dilantin*$_{US}$ anti-epileptic, frequently causes gingival hyperplasia and occasionally lupus erythematosus syndrome or erythema multiforme, action potentiated by **diazepam** and **aspirin**
Phyllocontin$_{GB,US}$	see **aminophylline**$_{GB,US}$
Physeptone$_{GB}$	see **methadone**$_{GB,US}$
Physostigmine$_{GB,US}$	anticholinesterase used as a miotic
Pilocarpine$_{GB,US}$	miotic
Pindolol$_{GB}$	(*Visken*$_{GB}$), beta-adrenergic blocker, hypotensive effect of general anaesthetics potentiated
Piperazine oestrone sulphate$_{GB,US}$	(*Harmogen*$_{GB}$) an oestrogen
Piriton$_{GB}$	see **chlopheniramine**$_{GB,US}$
Piroxicam$_{GB}$	(*Feldene*$_{GB}$), anti-inflammatory analgesic
Plaquenil$_{GB,US}$	see **hydroxychloroquine**$_{GB,US}$
Podophyllin$_{GB}$	used for treatment of warts
Poldine$_{GB}$	(*Nacton*$_{GB}$), antispasmodic used in peptic ulcer and spastic colon
Polymyxin$_{GB,US}$	antibiotic effective against Gram-negative organisms
Ponderax$_{GB}$	see **fenfluramine**$_{GB,US}$
Pondimin$_{US}$	see **fenfluramine**$_{US,GB}$
Ponstan$_{GB}$	see **mefanamic acid**
Potassium citrate$_{GB,US}$	for alkalinizing urine
Practolol$_{GB}$	(*Eraldin*$_{GB}$), beta-adrenergic blocker; serious side-effects limit its use to short-term treatment of dysrhythmias, hypotensive effects of general anaesthetics potentiated, oral erosions reported

Prazosin$_{GB,US}$ (*Minipress*$_{US}$, *Hypovase*$_{GB}$), potent vasodilator hypotensive agent, may potentiate hypotensive effect of general anaesthetics

Prednisolone$_{GB,US}$ corticosteroid, may suppress adrenals

Pregaday$_{GB}$ **iron + folate**

Prestim$_{GB}$ **timolol**$_{GB,US}$ + **bendrofluazide**$_{GB}$

Primaquine$_{GB,US}$ used to eradicate benign tertian malaria

Primidone$_{GB,US}$ (*Mysoline*$_{GB,US}$), for tonic, clonic, and partial seizures

Pro-banthine$_{GB,US}$ see **propantheline bromide**$_{GB,US}$

Probenecid$_{GB,US}$ (*Benemid*$_{GB,US}$), uricosuric agent; reduces renal excretion of **penicillin**; **aspirin** to be avoided

Procainamide$_{GB,US}$ (*Pronestyl*$_{GB}$), anti-arrhythmia agent, may cause lupus erythematosus syndrome

Procarbazine$_{GB,US}$ (*Natulan*$_{GB}$, *Matulane*$_{US}$), cytotoxic agent used in combination therapy for Hodgkin's disease, causes marrow depression

Prochlorperazine$_{GB,US}$ (*Stemetil*$_{GB}$) (*Compazine*$_{US}$), for schizophrenia and related psychoses

Procyclidine$_{GB,US}$ (*Kemadrin*$_{GB,US}$), anticholinergic drug used for Parkinsonism

Proguanil$_{GB}$ (*Paludrine*$_{GB}$), for prophylaxis against malaria, known to cause oral ulceration

Proloprim$_{US}$ see **trimethoprim**$_{US,GB}$

Promazine$_{GB}$ (*Sparine*$_{GB,US}$), for mild psychiatric disturbances in the elderly

Promethazine$_{GB,US}$ (*Phenergan*$_{GB,US}$), antihistamine

Propaderm$_{GB}$ see **beclomethasone dipropionate**$_{GB,US}$

Propantheline bromide$_{GB,US}$ (*Pro-banthine*$_{GB,US}$), anticholinergic agent, may cause a dry mouth

Propoxyphene napsylate$_{US}$ (*Darvocet-N*$_{US}$), medium-strength analgesic

Propranolol$_{GB,US}$ (*Inderal*$_{GB,US}$), beta-adrenergic blocker, hypotensive effect of general anaesthetics potentiated

Propylthiouracil$_{GB,US}$ used in the treatment of hyperthyroidism

Prostigmin$_{GB,US}$ see **neostigmine**$_{GB,US}$

Prothiaden$_{GB}$ see **dothiepin**$_{GB}$

Protriptyline$_{GB,US}$ tricyclic antidepressant with stimulant action, use LAs without **adrenaline**

Pyopen$_{GB,US}$	see **carbenicillin**
Pyrazinamide$_{GB}$	(*Zinamide*$_{GB}$), antituberculous antibiotic
Pyridostigmine$_{GB,US}$	(*Mestinon*$_{GB,US}$), anticholinesterase used for myasthenia gravis
Pyrimethamine$_{GB,US}$	(*Daraprim*$_{GB,US}$, *Fansidar*$_{GB}$), chemoprophylaxis of malaria
Pyrogastrone$_{GB}$	compound antacid
Questran$_{GB,US}$	see **cholestyramine**$_{GB,US}$
Quinidine$_{GB,US}$	used for supraventricular tachycardias, can cause oral erosions
Quinine$_{GB,US}$	used for malignant tertian malaria
Ranitidine$_{GB}$	(*Zantac*$_{GB}$), H2 receptor antagonist for treatment of dyspeptic conditions
Rapitard$_{GB}$	see **insulin**$_{GB,US}$
Rastinon$_{GB}$	see **tolbutamide**$_{GB,US}$
Rauwolfia$_{GB,US}$	(*Rautrax*$_{GB}$), hypotensive agent
Reserpine$_{GB,US}$	(*Serpasil*$_{GB,US}$), hypotensive agent
Rheumox$_{GB}$	see **azapropazone**$_{GB}$
Rifampicin$_{GB}$ **Rifampin**$_{US}$	first-line treatment of tuberculosis
Rivotril$_{GB}$	see **clonazepam**$_{GB,US}$
Rynacrom$_{GB}$	see **sodium cromoglycate**$_{GB}$, nasal insufflation
Rythmodan$_{GB}$	see **disopyramide**$_{GB,US}$
Salazopyrin$_{GB,US}$	see **sulphasalazine**$_{GB,US}$
Salbutamol$_{GB}$	(*Ventolin*$_{GB}$), beta-adrenoceptor stimulant for bronchospasm
Sandocal$_{GB}$	calcium preparation
Sanset$_{US}$	see **methysergide**$_{GB,US}$
Saventrine$_{GB}$	see **isoprenaline**$_{GB}$
Sectral$_{GB}$	see **acebutolol**$_{GB}$
Septin$_{GB}$	see **co-trimoxazole**$_{GB}$
Serc$_{GB}$	see **betahistine**$_{GB}$
Serenace$_{GB}$	see **haloperidol**$_{GB,US}$
Serenid$_{GB}$	see **oxazepam**$_{GB,US}$

Serpasil$_{GB,US}$	see **reserpine**$_{GB,US}$
Sinemet$_{GB,US}$	see **levodopa**$_{GB,US}$
Sodium amytal$_{GB}$	see **amylobarbitone sodium**$_{GB}$
Sodium aurothiomalate$_{GB}$	(*Myocrisin*$_{GB}$) for treatment of severe rheumatoid arthritis
Sodium cromoglycate$_{GB}$	(*Intal*$_{GB}$), cell membrane stabilizer used as prophylactic agent in asthma
Sodium fusidate$_{GB}$	(*Fucidine*$_{GB}$), narrow-spectrum antibiotic used for **penicillin**-resistant staphylococci
Sodium nitroprusside$_{GB,US}$	(*Nipride*$_{GB,US}$), used as intravenous infusion in hypertensive crises
Sodium valproate$_{GB}$	(*Epilim*$_{GB}$), used for tonic–clonic fits
Soframycin$_{GB}$	see **framycetin sulphate**$_{GB}$
Soneryl$_{GB}$	see **butobarbitone**$_{GB,US}$
Sotacor$_{GB}$	see **sotalol**$_{GB}$
Sotalol$_{GB}$	(*Sotacor*$_{GB}$), beta-adrenoceptor blocker, hypotensive effect of general anaesthetics potentiated
Sparine$_{GB,US}$	see **promazine**$_{GB}$
Spironolactone$_{GB,US}$	(*Aldactone*$_{GB,US}$), aldosterone antagonist; weak diuretic useful in oedematous states
Stanozolol$_{GB,US}$	(*Stromba*$_{GB}$), anabolic steroid
Stelabid$_{GB}$	**isopropamide**$_{GB,US}$ + **trifluoperazine**$_{GB,US}$
Stelazine$_{GB,US}$	see **trifluoperazine**$_{GB,US}$
Stemetil$_{GB}$	see **prochlorperazine**$_{GB,US}$
Sterculia$_{GB}$	(*Normacol*$_{GB}$), bulk laxative
Stilboestrol$_{GB}$	female sex hormone used in treatment of prostatic carcinoma
Strepsils$_{GB}$	antiseptic lozenges
Streptomycin$_{GB}$	first-line drug for tuberculosis; serious side-effects, ototoxicity, and nephrotoxicity
Stromba$_{GB}$	see **stanozolol**$_{GB,US}$
Stugeron$_{GB}$	see **cinnarizine**$_{GB}$
Sulindac$_{GB,US}$	(*Clinoril*$_{GB,US}$), anti-inflammatory analgesic
Sulthiame$_{GB}$	(*Ospolot*$_{GB}$), for myoclonic seizures and hyperkinesia, may cause paraesthesia of face
Sulphacetamide$_{GB,US}$	sulphonamide for eye infections
Sulphadiazine$_{GB,US}$	sulphonamide used for meningococcal meningitis
Sulphadimidine$_{GB}$	sulphonamide for urinary tract infections

Sulphamethizole$_{GB,US}$	sulphonamide for urinary tract infections
Sulphasalazine$_{GB,US}$	(*Salazopyrine*$_{GB,US}$), for treatment of ulcerative colitis
Sulphinpyrazone$_{GB,US}$	(*Anturan*$_{GB,US}$), anti-platelet drug used for prophylaxis after myocardial infarctions
Surmontil$_{GB,US}$	see **trimipramine**$_{GB,US}$
Sustac$_{GB}$	see **glyceryl trinitrate**$_{GB,US}$
Symmetrel$_{GB,US}$	see **amantadine**$_{GB,US}$
Synacthen$_{GB}$	see **tetracosactrin**$_{GB}$

Tagamet$_{GB,US}$	see **cimetidine**$_{GB,US}$
Talampicillin$_{GB}$	(*Talpen*$_{GB}$), ester of **ampicillin** rapidly absorbed from the gut, may effect adsorption of oral contraceptives
Talpen$_{GB}$	see **talampicillin**$_{US,GB}$
Talwin$_{US}$	see **pentazocine**$_{US,GB}$
Tamoxifen$_{GB,US}$	(*Nolvadex*$_{GB,US}$), anti-oestrogen for breast cancer
Tandearil$_{US}$	see **oxyphenbutazone**$_{GB,US}$
Tanderil$_{GB}$	see **oxyphenbutazone**$_{GB,US}$
Tegopen$_{US}$	see **cloxacillin**
Tegretol$_{GB,US}$	see **carbamazepine**$_{GB,US}$
Temazepam$_{GB}$	(*Normison*$_{GB}$), hypnotic and sedative
Temgesic$_{GB}$	see **buprenorphine**$_{GB}$
Tenoretic$_{GB}$	**atenolol**$_{GB}$ + **chlorthalidone**$_{GB,US}$
Tenormin$_{GB}$	see **atenolol**$_{GB}$
Tensilon$_{GB,US}$	see **edrophonium chloride**$_{GB,US}$
Tenuate$_{GB,US}$	see **diethylpropion**$_{GB,US}$
Terbutaline$_{GB,US}$	(*Bricanyl*$_{GB,US}$), beta-adrenoceptor stimulant for bronchospasm
Terramycin$_{GB,US}$	see **oxytetracycline**$_{GB,US}$
Tetracosactrin$_{GB}$	(*Synactren*$_{GB}$) adrenal stimulant
Tetracycline$_{GB,US}$	broad-spectrum antibiotic useful in treatment of rickettsia and mycoplasma
Theophylline$_{GB,US}$	(*Nuelin*$_{GB}$), xanthine derivative used for bronchospasm
Thioguanine$_{GB,US}$	(*Lanvis*$_{GB}$), antimetabolite for acute leukaemias, causes marrow depression
Thioridazine$_{GB,US}$	(*Melleril*$_{GB,US}$), antipsychotic drug
Thiotepa$_{GB,US}$	alkylating agent for malignant effusions

Thyroxine$_{GB,US}$ — (*Eltroxin*$_{GB}$, *Synthroid*$_{US}$), thyroid hormone for replacement therapy in hypothyroidism

Timolol$_{GB,US}$ — (*Blocadven*$_{GB}$) beta-adrenoceptor blocker for hypertension and angina, hypotensive effects of general anaesthetics potentiated

Tobramycin$_{GB,US}$ — aminoglycoside for treatment of pseudomonas infections

Tofranil$_{GB,US}$ — see **imipramine**$_{GB,US}$

Tolbutamide$_{GB,US}$ — (*Rastinon*$_{GB}$), sulphonylurea used as oral hypoglycaemic in diabetes, potentiated by **aspirin**; has been known to cause oral erosions

Trandate$_{GB}$ — see **labetalol**$_{GB}$

Tranexamic acid$_{GB}$ — (*Cyklokapron*$_{GB}$), antifibrinolytic agent used for haemorrhage after prostatectomy

Tranxene$_{GB,US}$ — see **clorazepate**$_{GB}$

Tranylcypromine$_{GB,US}$ — (*Parnate*$_{GB,US}$), MAOI for depressive illness, **amphetamine, ephedrine,** and narcotic analgesics to be avoided

Trasicor$_{GB}$ — see **oxprenolol**$_{GB}$

Trasidrex$_{GB}$ — **oxprenolol**$_{GB}$ + **cyclopenthiazide**$_{GB}$

Trasylol$_{GB}$ — see **aprotinin**$_{GB}$

Triamcinolone$_{GB,US}$ — (*Adcortyl*$_{GB}$, *Kenalog*$_{US}$), corticosteroid

Triamterene$_{GB,US}$ — (*Dyazide*$_{GB,US}$, *Dytac*$_{GB}$), oedema and potassium conservaton with thiazide and loop diuretics

Triazolam$_{GB}$ — (*Halcion*$_{GB}$), hypnotic and sedative

Trifluoperazine$_{GB,US}$ — (*Stelazine*$_{GB,US}$), for schizophrenia and related psychoses

Trimeprazine$_{GB,US}$ — (*Vallergan*$_{GB}$), antipruritic agent

Trimethoprim$_{GB,US}$ — (*Monotrim*$_{GB}$, *Proloprim*$_{US}$), broad-spectrum antibiotic

Trimipramine$_{GB,US}$ — (*Surmontil*$_{GB,US}$), tricyclic antidepressant with sedative properties, use LAs without **adrenaline**

Tripotassium dicitratobismuthate$_{GB}$ — (*De-Nol*$_{GB}$), ulcer healing agent

Triptizol$_{GB}$ — see **amitriptyline**$_{GB,US}$

Tryptophan$_{GB,US}$ — tricyclic antidepressant, use LAs without **adrenaline**

Urispas$_{US,GB}$	see **flavoxate**$_{US\ GB}$
Urolucosil$_{GB}$	see **sulphamethizole**$_{GB,US}$
Ursodeoxycholic acid$_{GB}$	for dissolution of cholesterol gallstones
Valium$_{GB,US}$	see **diazepam**$_{GB,US}$
Vallergan$_{GB}$	see **trimeprazine**$_{GB,US}$
Valproic acid$_{US}$	(*Depokene*$_{US}$), used for petit mal
Vancomycin$_{GB,US}$	bactericidal antibiotic; used for the treatment of pseudomembranous colitis
Vascardin$_{GB}$	see **isosorbide**$_{GB,US}$
Vasopressin$_{GB,US}$	antidiuretic hormone; treatment for diabetes insipidus
Velbe$_{GB}$	see **vinblastine**$_{GB,US}$
Velosef$_{GB,US}$	see **cephradine**$_{GB,US}$
Ventolin$_{GB}$	see **salbutamol**$_{GB}$
Verapamil$_{GB}$	(*Cordilox*$_{GB}$), used for supraventricular arrhythmias
Vinblastine$_{GB,US}$	(*Velbe*$_{GB}$), vinca alkaloid; management of lymphomas, causes marrow depression
Vincristine$_{GB,US}$	(*Oncovin*$_{GB,US}$), vinca alkaloid; major drug in management of lymphomas and leukaemia, causes marrow depression
Viskaldix$_{GB}$	**pindolol**$_{GB}$ + **clopamide**$_{GB}$
Voltarol$_{GB}$	see **diclofenac**$_{GB}$
Warfarin$_{GB,US}$	(*Marevan*$_{GB}$, *Coumadin*$_{US}$), anticoagulant, potentiated by **aspirin, mefenamic** acid, **metronidazole**
Welldorm$_{GB}$	see **dichloralphenazone**$_{GB,US}$
Xylometazoline$_{GB,US}$	(*Otrivine*$_{GB}$, *Otrivin*$_{US}$), nasal decongestant, to be avoided in patients on MAOIs
Zaditen$_{GB}$	see **ketotifen**$_{GB}$
Zarontin$_{GB,US}$	see **ethosuximide**$_{GB,US}$
Zinacef$_{GB}$	see **cefuroxime**$_{GB}$
Zinamide$_{GB}$	see **pyrazinamide**$_{GB}$
Zyloprim$_{US}$	see **allopurinol**$_{GB,US}$
Zyloric$_{GB}$	see **allopurinol**$_{GB,US}$